Specialist Foster Family Care: A Normalizing Experience

THE CHILD & YOUTH SERVICES SERIES

- *Institutional Abuse of Children & Youth*, edited by Ranae Hanson
- *Youth Participation & Experiential Education*, edited by Daniel Conrad and Diane Hedin
- *Legal Reforms Affecting Child & Youth Services*, edited by Gary B. Melton
- *Social Skills Training for Children and Youth*, edited by Craig W. LeCroy
- *Adolescent Substance Abuse: A Guide to Prevention and Treatment*, edited by Richard Isralowitz and Mark Singer
- *Young Girls: A Portrait of Adolescence*, by Gisela Konopka
- *Adolescents, Literature, and Work with Youth*, co-edited by J. Pamela Weiner and Ruth M. Stein
- *Residential Group Care in Community Context: Implications From the Israeli Experience*, edited by Zvi Eisikovits and Jerome Beker
- *Helping Delinquents Change: A Treatment Manual of Social Learning Approaches*, by Jerome Stumphauzer
- *Qualitative Research and Evaluation in Group Care*, edited by Rivka Eisikovits and Yitzhak Kashti
- *The Black Adolescent Parent*, edited by Stanley F. Battle
- *Developmental Group Care of Children and Youth: Concepts and Practice*, by Henry W. Maier
- *Assaultive Youth: Responding to Physical Assaultiveness in Residential, Community and Health Care Settings*, edited by Joel Kupfersmid and Roberta Monkman
- *Family Perspectives in Child and Youth Services*, edited by David H. Olson
- *Transitioning Exceptional Children and Youth into the Community: Research and Practice*, edited by Ennio Cipani
- *Helping the Youthful Offender: Individual and Group Therapies That Work*, by William B. Lewis
- *Specialist Foster Family Care: A Normalizing Experience*, edited by Joe Hudson and Burt Galaway

Specialist Foster Family Care: A Normalizing Experience

Joe Hudson
Burt Galaway
Editors

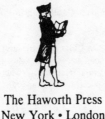

The Haworth Press
New York • London

Specialist Foster Family Care: A Normalizing Experience has also been published as *Child & Youth Services*, Volume 12, Numbers 1/2 1989.

The Haworth Press, Inc., 10 Alice Street, Binghamton, NY 13904-1580.
EUROSPAN/Haworth, 3 Henrietta Street, London WC2E 8LU England

Library of Congress Cataloging-in-Publication Data

Specialist foster family care.
    Published also as v. 12, no. 1/2 of Child & youth services.
    Includes bibliographical references.
    1. Child psychotherapy—Residential treatment. 2. Mentally ill children—Rehabilitation. 3. Foster home care—Psychological aspects. I. Hudson, Joe.
II. Galaway, Burt.
RJ504.5.S65 1989   618.92'8914   89-15648
ISBN 0-86656-939-1

Specialist Foster Family Care: A Normalizing Experience

CONTENTS

CONCLUSION

ABOUT THE EDITORS

Burt Galaway, PhD, MA, is Professor at the School of Social Work, University of Minnesota in Minneapolis. His social work practice experience has been in child welfare, corrections, and victim service agencies; he has done research in the areas of restitution, criminal justice, spouse battering, crime victim offender mediation, and child welfare. In 1982 Dr. Galaway was the recipient of a research fellowship from the New Zealand National Research Advisory Council and spent twelve months as a senior research fellow with the New Zealand Department of Justice. Dr. Galaway is author or co-author of several books, including *Medication in Criminal Justice: Victim, Offenders and Communities* (1988), *Social Work Processes* (1975, 1979, 1984), *Public Acceptance of Restitution as an Alternative Imprisonment for Property Offenders: A Survey* (1984), *Considering the Victim* (1975), *Community Corrections: Selected Readings* (1976), *Restitution and Criminal Justice* (1977), *Offender Restitution in Theory and Action* (1978), *Victims, Offenders and Alternative Sanctions* (1980), and *Perspectives on Crime Victims* (1981), as well as numerous articles.

Joe Hudson, PhD, MSW, is Associate Professor at the Faculty of Social Welfare, The University of Calgary in Edmonton, Alberta, Canada. His work experience has been in adult and juvenile corrections, victim services, and auditing. Dr. Hudson has served with the Minnesota Department of Corrections and the Office of the Auditor General of Canada. He has done research in the areas of restitution and community service work order programs. Dr. Hudson has served as editor of the outstanding achievement award from the Canadian Evaluation Society. His publications include *Justice As Fairness* (1981), *perspectives on Crime Victims* (1980), *The Serious Juvenile Offender* (1977), *Offender Restitution in Theory and Action* (1978), *Restitution in Criminal Justice* (1977), *Community Corrections: A Book of Readings* (1976), *Considering the Victim* (1975), as well as numerous articles.

Foreword

Nearly three decades ago, as a beginning social worker in a private child welfare agency, I was involved in the establishment of a new, "specialized foster care" program for emotionally disturbed children and youth. It was an exciting time, as my colleagues and I sought to develop a program focusing on foster care as a therapeutic modality, rather than a custodial service, for young people and their families. In this process, we struggled with many issues, in areas such as definition of specialized foster care; structure, components, and effectiveness of the program; private-public partnership; recruitment, training, and retention of foster parents; participation of biological parents in the helping process; and clarification of roles of social workers, foster parents, and other members of the treatment team.

These issues, and the sense of excitement of long ago, came back to me in full force as I read this book. More importantly, however, I realized that we have come a long way in the area of foster care programming—and particularly in respect to what the editors call *specialist foster family care*. While the issues identified decades ago are still alive and well, the contributors to this volume offer a penetrating examination of possible solutions and a careful description of the state of the art in the field, from the American, British, and Canadian perspectives.

Especially impressive is the clear and consistent emphasis on specialist foster care—whatever term may be preferred by individual authors—as a viable and vital form of community care for children and youth experiencing a range of problems and needs. Moreover, the authors explore and clarify the therapeutic potential of the foster family; the supports necessary to realize such potential on behalf of each young person; the diversity of program models and strategies; the establishment of specialized foster care services in public child welfare agencies; and the application to a range of cli-

xiii

ent groups, including autistic, handicapped, and sexually abused children.

As a result, this volume makes an excellent and practical contribution to the literature. It should be read widely; its ideas and experiences will be of interest to many in the human services. Its insights will be useful to anyone concerned with permanency planning and family preservation in general, and the use of foster care as a rehabilitative and growth-producing tool in particular. Program planners and administrators will find especially valuable various chapters on program design, implementation, and evaluation.

The volume thus has much to offer that can be put to immediate use in different agencies and programs. In addition, it is forward-looking, in that the contributors highlight issues and challenges that must receive further attention as specialist foster family care evolves as a distinctive modality. These issues are thoughtfully delineated by the editors in the concluding chapter, particularly in relation to comparative analysis of contrasting models and their components, uses, and outcomes; strengthening the involvement of birth parents; clarifying the relationship of specialized foster family care to permanency planning; and extending foster family care services to additional populations, including adults. There is also the need to consider more explicitly the relevance of various models for minority families and children who, at least in the United States are overrepresented in the foster care population.

The book will undoubtedly stimulate consideration of these issues, as agencies seek to strengthen or expand their services to families with children in out-of-home placement or at risk of such placement. In so doing, agencies should pay attention to an even more basic issue that is implicit throughout the book but not explored in depth: the need for a thorough reexamination of traditional foster family care and its role in contemporary society.

Many of the authors in this volume refer to the changing nature of children and youth entering traditional foster care. As they suggest, there is substantial evidence that most young people in care are increasingly "difficult," "troubled," and "troubling"; from "disorganized" and "multi-problem" families; and traumatized by experiences of abuse and neglect. Yet, it is well known that specialized programs reach only a small proportion of these youngsters. In light of all this, we need to raise some questions: Should we see specialist foster family care as a service for a selected few? Should we think of it as an *alternative* to traditional foster family care, or as *the* modality required by most—if not all—young people in care? Can we use what we are learning through specialized models to enrich all foster care programs?

These questions may betray a utopian perspective—but they need to be considered to counteract the trend toward separating or distancing specialized foster family care models from more "traditional" forms of foster care or from the field of child welfare as a whole. Such a trend is evident in this book, as it is in the world of practice. Unless we question its rationale, we may well face the emergence of two separate and unequal foster care systems—an elite system for the few in private agencies and a poorly supported and ineffective system for the many in public agencies. Is this what we want? If not, how can we avoid such an outcome? Perhaps another conference and another book are called for to explore and resolve these questions.

Anthony N. Maluccio
School of Social Work
University of Connecticut

INTRODUCTION

Chapter 1

Specialist Fostering:
Resources and Activities

Joe Hudson
Burt Galaway

ABSTRACT. Specialist foster family care is a new programming thrust; we lack essential information regarding program resources, program activities, and program outcomes. Conceptual models will offer descriptions of the resources, activities, and outcomes of the specialized foster care schemes. Resources include types of youth and children served, types of specialist foster parents recruited and trained for service, role and responsibility of social workers, and involvement of birth parents in the programs. Activities need to be specified, including recruitment and licensure activities, placement activities, and the nature of the programming which occurs in placement. Specialist foster family care appears to be a viable form of services to children and youth, but its future development will depend on ability to specify program resources and program activities.

Joe Hudson is Professor on the Faculty of Social Welfare, University of Calgary (Edmonton Division), 8625 – 112th Street, #300, Edmonton, Alberta T6G 1K8 Canada. Burt Galaway is Professor at the School of Social Work, University of Minnesota, 224 Church Street S. E., #400, Minneapolis, MN 55455.

1

Foster care programming in North America dates back to the mid-nineteenth century and the work of Charles Loring Brace, but only in the past two decades have we seen significant developments in treatment, therapeutic or specialized foster care programming. This type of programming evolved in the United States in two major stages (Bryant, 1981; 1983). The first stage covered the 1950s and early 1960s, when specialized foster care programs were used as supplements to psychiatric hospitals and residential treatment centers, aimed at providing a transitional experience for youth returning to the community.

The second stage of development has been traced by Bryant to the deinstitutionalization movement of the late 1960s, with special fostering schemes being used as alternatives to institutional placement. Further developments in specialized fostering arrangements have continued over the last several years with international conferences devoted to the topic, an evolving professional organization and the establishment of several hundred programs in North America. This book is further evidence of the growing interest in special fostering programs operating as both the context and means for dealing with persons in need of family-based services and who, for whatever reason, cannot remain with their birth families.

This book is intended as an introduction to the rapidly growing field of specialist fostering. The chapters identify critical issues bearing on specialized fostering arrangements, trace policy developments, and present program examples. Most of these chapters were initially presented as papers at the First North American Conference on Treatment Foster Care held in 1987 in Minneapolis. This conference was jointly sponsored by five Minnesota specialist fostering agencies for the purpose of examining specialized foster care as part of the continuum of services for children and youth.

The book is organized in three major sections: program perspectives and principles, program issues, and approaches for delivering services. This introductory chapter describes some key program elements and issues associated with specialist fostering arrangements and relates these to the chapters that follow. Our concluding chapter reconsiders a number of these matters and looks forward to future needs in policy, program, and research developments.

OVERVIEW OF THE BOOK

Chapters 2 and 3 by Nancy Hazel and Pamela Meadowcroft respectively, open Part I of the collection; they present broad perspectives on the practice principles incorporated in specialized or treatment foster care and identify significant issues. Hazel, founder of the Kent Family Placement Program in Canterbury, England, describes key ingredients of the Kent Project, provides a retrospective look at foster care developments in England over the past two decades and identifies matters on which further work is required. Meadowcroft focuses on North American developments and mirrors matters raised by Hazel. Both authors point to the promise specialist fostering schemes hold for young persons who would otherwise be placed in institutional care.

This theme is addressed again in Chapter 4 by Peter Smith who enlarges on the theoretical basis for the Kent Family Placement Service and the way these principles have been incorporated in program practices. The importance of identity development in adolescence is highlighted by Smith, particularly in terms of the role played by significant persons, such as biological parents and siblings. The crucial importance of building and maintaining links between youth in care and their birth families is then a recurring theme in the papers that follow. Peter Forsythe deals in detail with the theme of family connectedness in Chapter 5 and presents a challenge for specialist fostering programs to work as extensions of the biological family, not as isolated alternatives to it.

Chapter 6 by Mary McColgan gives an historical review of the evolution of foster care in Northern Ireland. Her case study of that country closely resembles significant milestones in the development of foster care in Canada and the United States. Only recently in Northern Ireland have specialist fostering schemes developed to serve youth in place of institutional settings and, as in the United States, the early programs have been pioneered by the private sector. McColgan notes the importance of programs sharing information on their structure, experience and results so that improved services can be delivered to the clients served.

The eight chapters in Part II move to consider specific program matters including characteristics of persons served, emancipation issues, training, and program implementation. Chapters 7, 8, and 9, by Emily Jean McFadden, Susan Whitelaw Downs, and Clarice Rosen, respectively, deal with schemes serving special categories of young persons, including autistic children, youth with histories of sexual abuse, and those with developmental disabilities. Chapter 10, by Emily Jean McFadden, Dale Rice, Patricia Ryan, and Bruce Warren, deals in detail with the variety of matters associated with the emancipation process of youth leaving care. These authors underscore the important role played by families in helping young people establish a clear sense of identity by mirroring back a sense of who they are. The point is made that multiple foster family placements can have the effect of "a wilderness of mirrors" reflecting back fragmented images to the youth.

Placement disruption may result from lack of training provided to foster parents; Chapter 11 by Juanita Baker presents a description of a training approach used in Florida. Chapter 12 by Brad Bryant, Fred Simmens, and Mary McKee presents different perspectives on implementing specialist foster care programming in Missouri. As these authors note, specialized foster care programs established in the United States have generally been started by private agencies, and special challenges are presented for attempts at implementing programs within a large public agency. Three different perspectives are offered on the implementation effort in Missouri—the viewpoints of a state administrator (Simmens), local project worker (McKee), and private agency consultant (Bryant). Chapter 13, by Brian Charbonneau and Ziona Kaplan, describes group work with biological parents of children being served in a specialist foster care program. In Chapter 14, Ziona Kaplan and Edith Fein deal with the place of specialist fostering on the continuum of services that should be available to youth requiring out-of-home care.

A number of the issues identified in Part II are dealt with in the context of the program descriptions contained in Part III. These six chapters describe programs operating under both public and private auspices in England, Canada, and the United States. While these programs operate in different ways and serve persons with different problems in living, they illustrate ways in which many of the significant issues identified in earlier chapters can be addressed. For example, Chapter 15 by Grace Sisto and Myra Maker illustrates the importance of including biological parents in a service program by providing care for teenage mothers and their babies so as to strengthen the bond between them. The PATH program described by Michael Peterson illustrates the role of foster parents in directing a specialist fostering agency.

The importance of emancipation services for youth leaving care is emphasized in Chapter 17 by Christopher Kelley and James Carruth, while Chapter 18 on the Human Service Associates program emphasizes a service philosophy of least restrictive alternative and the provision of opportunities to youth to accomplish developmental tasks and develop competencies in living. Chapter 19 by Ruben Orenstein on the New Brunswick, Canada, province-wide program provides a complement to the earlier chapter by Bryant and his colleagues on the implementation of a statewide specialist program in Missouri. While most of the chapters deal with services for children and youth, family-based services can also be provided to older persons; Chapter 20 by Leigh Jones provides a description of such a program in Hampshire, England.

A major question confronting specialist fostering arrangements is the manner and extent to which they differ from traditional foster care programs. Is specialist foster care simply old wine in new bottles, a new name for what has long been preached, if not practiced, in foster care? Authors of the chapters in this volume generally take the position that specialist fostering is qualitatively different from traditional foster care. Clearly, however, all forms of family care have in common the notion that families can best serve as a principle environmental source of social support in the lives of people. Through family relationships and social interaction, children and youth can be provided with necessary affective, cognitive, and instrumental resources to get about the work of growing and developing with a sense of permanence and continuity. How these efforts are carried out may vary from program to program.

We lack detailed, current information on specialist schemes operating in different jurisdictions. Only limited demographic program data is available from North American surveys completed by Bryant (1983) and Snodgrass and Bryant (1984), along with the results of a British survey reported by Shaw and Hipgrave (1983) and Pamela

Meadowcroft's survey done at the Minnesota Conference and reported in Chapter 3.

Brad Bryant's 1980 survey covered eight specialist fostering programs, while the Snodgrass and Bryant survey is based on questionnaire responses from 48 treatment foster care programs operating in March-April 1984 in North America. Shaw and Hipgrave's survey reports information on 45 specialist fostering programs operating throughout the United Kingdom in 1982, while Meadowcroft's survey of 400 attendees at the First North American Conference in 1987 identified over a hundred programs in the United States and Canada.

The North American surveys report programs operating in a large number of states and provinces, most by private nonprofit agencies and most relatively recently implemented. Meadowcroft reports, for example, that only half of the one hundred programs represented at the 1987 Minnesota conference existed prior to 1985 and fewer than 10 percent had been operating for more than 10 years. Approximately two thirds of the programs identified by Snodgrass and Bryant served youth as an alternative to institutional placement and most were small, with approximately three quarters of those identified serving 30 or fewer clients. The United Kingdom survey reported similar results, finding that over 80 percent of the schemes had been in operation for five years or less, with over two thirds serving 13 or fewer placements.

Besides demographic characteristics of specialist fostering arrangements, key programming characteristics can be identified, along with some of the issues and concerns associated with the development of this relatively new program venture. For our purposes, major program ingredients can be identified as they emerge from a description of program resources and activities.

PROGRAM RESOURCES

Major types of resources used in specialist fostering programs are people — the clients or persons served, foster parents, and other helping persons, usually social workers, associated with the program. In those cases where the specialist foster program operates as a private agency, additional resources are often provided by the public agencies making referrals, as well as by ancillary service providers such as educators and therapists. While the major sets of participants in these schemes can be found in more traditional foster care practices, they are often seen as differing with respect to the expectations held for foster parents, the status associated with their role, and the severity of problems presented by the youth served.

Youth and Children Served

Children and youth served by specialist fostering programs are seen as high-risk, having a variety of problems in living that make them hard to place and maintain in traditional foster homes. Emily McFadden, for example, describes work with the sexually abused child in specialized foster care, Clarice Rosen with autistic children, Susan Downs with retarded and physically handicapped youth, and Grace Sisto and Myra Maker with adolescent mothers and their babies. In short, specialist foster care programs tend to support the point made by Nancy Hazel that no person should be seen as unsuitable for family placement.

The characteristics of persons served by these fostering schemes will likely relate to the length and type of services provided. Are specialist placements relatively long-term, ending with the youth's emancipation to independent living, or do they serve youth for a relatively brief period of time before youth are returned to their natural families? And if children do spend relatively brief periods of time in specialized care, does this mean they are moved in and out of care? Should specialist foster care be reserved for children and youth requiring long-term, relatively permanent placement? If so, what are the implications for the program, especially in terms of working with the biological family? These are important questions on which we have only limited information.

In terms of length of care, the information available tends to indicate that specialist programs provide relatively short term care. The Snodgrass and Bryant survey found the average length of placement for youth discharged in 1983 from 34 programs to be 14 months (1984, p. 33), while almost three quarters of the 43 schemes surveyed by Shaw and Hipgrave in the United Kingdom served children and youth for between six months and two years (1983, p. 140).

Many of the programs covered in this book are described as placement alternatives to institutional congregate care settings and operate as institutional alternatives in two ways. One way is for the specialist scheme to serve as an alternative placement to congregate care facilities; the other is for the specialist program to serve children and youth as a transition from such facilities. Presumably, the aim is to shorten the length of time in institutional care if one cannot eliminate it entirely.

Any particular specialist program may operate in either or both ways, depending on the source of referrals for the program. Key questions then arise about the bases on which referral decisions are made, both in terms of the amount and type of information collected and the way information is assessed and used to make decisions about persons in care. A large proportion of specialist foster care programs are run by private agencies with key decisions about program referrals made by officials in local, state, or provincial governments. There is reason to be concerned about the amount and type of information used by child welfare officials, the way this information is collected, and the criteria against which it is assessed in making significant decisions about persons in care (Stein, Gambrill, & Wiltse, 1978).

The possibility arises out of treatment foster programs operating to widen and deepen the net of state intervention and control over youth served. Peter Forsythe raises this concern in Chapter 5. The history of the community corrections or deinstitutionalization movement in the juvenile justice system lends credence to such a possibility. State restrictiveness will be increased if specialist foster programs operate as supplements to traditional foster care or in-home care. Some indirect evidence is available on this from the Snodgrass and Bryant survey on 34 treatment foster programs. Their data show that approximately one-third of youth admitted to the specialist programs in 1983 entered from their own homes or homes of relatives, and almost an additional one-fifth from regular foster care (1984, p. 22). At the same time, two-thirds of the surveyed programs set as their purpose to serve as alternatives to institutions and one-third to serve as alternatives to regular foster care (1984, p. 25).

Using specialist foster care as an alternative to traditional foster care or to in-home care may not, from one perspective, be problematic. In this view specialist foster care programs deliver a richer array of services than those available in more traditional foster care or even in the youth's home. As Nancy Hazel notes, care should be seen as a positive experience. The experience of youth moving between the specialist home and the birth family home can be one of providing opportunities for growth and development.

The propensity of total institutional settings to severely damage the development of young people and the responsibility to reduce these damaging effects by using specialist foster family resources for youth who would otherwise go into institutional care must be recognized in considering who should best be served by specialist foster care programs. Total institutions violate most severely the principle of normalization, and therefore greater effort should be given to reducing the number of children placed in such restrictive settings. From this view public decision makers should establish procedures to help ensure that youth actually served by specialist foster care programs would, in their absence, have otherwise been placed in institutions, not drained off from in-home care. The question needing to be addressed is whether specialist foster care programs can, in fact, provide the necessary services to this target group of youth. Can these homes retain these youth in care and delivery the types of services claimed, thus serving as a viable alternative to institutions?

To answer those questions we need well-designed evaluations aimed at assessing the relative benefits of specialist foster care and congregate care institutions. Ideally, this would take the form of an experimental design in which referrals to the treatment institution would be randomly assigned to either the institution or the specialist fostering scheme. The persons served could be followed during program exposure and on completion of the service with comparisons made on measures of efficiency and effectiveness. This type of study is timely, ethically appropriate, and likely to provide useful information for child welfare decision making. The respective comparison programs are quite amenable to precise definition and, so long as the persons to be randomly assigned would have received the more intrusive treatment, allocation to the alternative specialist fostering program is ethically appropriate. Conducting such a study in several jurisdictions with a variety of specialist programs and institutions could help give greater confidence to the results and provide information as to the most appropriate client resources for specialist foster family programs.

Specialist Foster Parents

Specialist foster parents are an essential program resource. All of the chapters emphasize the central role played by foster parents in delivering services to youth in care. Nancy Hazel and Peter Smith, for example, emphasize the principle of egalitarianism, so that foster parents, along with youth in care and their families, are regarded as equal in status to other program professionals. Peter Forsythe underscores this point by suggesting that the relationship between specialist and traditional foster care is analogous to that between a residential treatment center and an orphanage. Meadowcroft pursues this analogy by noting that family care is residential care at its best.

Most programs set requirements of fostering experience, education, and pre-service training. When prior fostering experience is used as a program requirement, however, it may well have implications for traditional foster programs by exacerbating the difficulties experienced in recruiting and maintaining foster homes. An important question then becomes the extent to which specialist fostering programs are creaming the most experienced and skillful foster parents from regular fostering schemes. Other questions have to do with the extent to which training requirements result in delivering enhanced services, as well as the extent to which training is related to the length of time parents remain as service providers.

Much of the training given to specialist foster parents places heavy emphasis on behavioral management, communications skills, and the developmental needs of young persons. An example of a detailed training approach used by the Florida Institute of Technology is given in Chapter 11 by Juanita Baker. In addition, more specialized and targeted types of training are being offered in specialist programs to address the particular needs of specific types of youth. Examples of training programs for dealing with the sexually abused child and emancipating youths are contained, respectively, in Chapter 7 by Emily Jean McFadden and Chapter 10 by McFadden and her colleagues. An interesting question then arises around the extent to which training efforts conflict with the principle of egalitarianism in the daily life of any program, especially in those cases where social workers in the program are the primary training source. Specialist foster parents may be seen as needing to be trained by agency social workers while failing to appreciate that the converse situation may be just as crucial.

The increased level of compensation provided to treatment parents is another resource characteristic of specialist fostering schemes. The 42 agencies on which Snodgrass and Bryant collected information during 1984 found that the mean monthly payment to foster parents was slightly over $500. Pamela Meadowcroft suggests in Chapter 3 that useful guidelines for establishing payment rates for treatment parents is simply to double the local rate paid to traditional foster parents. While the different chapters have little to say about the actual rates charged by the different programs, they all note that enhanced payment levels are provided and, in turn, relate this to the heavy demands placed on specialist foster parents, the special difficulties they experience in dealing with the exceptional children placed, and the eligibility and training requirements. Will enhanced pay assist in recruiting effective specialist foster parents? The survey data reported in Chapter 8 by Susan Whitelaw Downs found that increasing payment rates for foster parents serving retarded and physically handicapped children may have a positive effect on the number of persons willing to take on the special demands of caring for these young people.

Limited financial resources available to the state, along with the high cost of institutional care and the increased frequency of two-income families in our society, will put increased pressure on public officials to reallocate the dollars available to provide enhanced levels of compensation for specialist foster parents. The fact is that fewer families are likely to be available to volunteer their parenting skills as foster parents. The career option of both parents being paid at competitive rates for their services may increase the availability of parents willing to take on the special demands of dealing with troubled youth.

Social Workers

Another category of resources used in specialist schemes are social workers or other types of professional helpers employed by the program to assist foster parents in providing care. Each of the programs described in these chapters employs social workers or other professionals to work with foster parents and, in each, reduced caseloads are a common feature. Smaller caseloads are designed to help ensure that social workers are closely involved with treatment parents, children, and natural parents in meeting service standards.

The fact that a large proportion of specialist fostering programs are operated as private agencies and accept referrals from public authorities means that two social workers will be involved with youth who are placed — the worker employed by the private specialist program and the public agency worker responsible for making referrals, monitoring ongoing progress, and reporting to other social welfare authorities. This dual set of roles is likely to add to the complexity of specialist schemes and underscore the importance of clearly defining the rights and responsibilities of each party with respect to the youth, the birth parents, and the specialist foster parents. A similar situation is likely to exist in public agencies responsible for operating specialist fostering programs with different sets of workers responsible for handling different tasks associated with the placement — recruiting and licensing homes, referring and placing youth, monitoring and managing service delivery.

Birth Parents

Birth parents of youth in care are increasingly being seen as an important resource to be tapped by specialist schemes in work with the youth. In some programs the resources of the biological family are pooled with those of the specialist foster home in a partnership arrangement for working with youth in care. But more than rhetoric is needed. Careful and sustained effort must be given in specialist programs to encourage and support links between children and their parents, and systematic monitoring activities need to be conducted to ensure that program practices mirror program principles.

PROGRAM ACTIVITIES

Specialist foster care programs generally engage in four primary types of service activities—recruiting and licensing treatment homes, preparing for placement, implementing service plans, and discharge and follow-up.

Recruitment and Licensure

A variety of practices are commonly used to recruit parents, including newspaper advertisements, radio and television announcements, speeches to community groups, consultation with community leaders, and work with foster parents are prime recruitment sources. In Chapter 3, Pamela Meadowcroft describes the small number of families actually licensed as specialist parents compared to the large number initially attracted to seek information about taking up such work. This dramatic attrition means that recruitment must be ongoing and requires sustained attention and effort.

Placement

Three sets of activities are commonly carried out in specialist schemes following the referral of youth for placement. These amount to identifying available homes and making a tentative match, exchanging information between the youth and potential specialist foster parents, and preparing a service agreement or treatment contract.

While considerable effort has been directed at identifying the characteristics of successful foster parents and determining variables to be used in matching parents with youth, little success has been demonstrated. Many different kinds of people can likely perform well as foster parents and, given the multiplicity of variables associated with the different parties to a fostering arrangement, it is probably fruitless for programs to spend time and money collecting a lot of information for use in elaborate matching procedures. More important is the amount and type of information exchanged between social workers, potential specialist foster parents, biological parents, and the youth to be placed, including information about the reasons for the placement, services to be provided, and the goals to be achieved. The importance of pre-placement visits and opportunities they provide for the parties to collect and assess information in making placement decisions are noted in several of the chapters.

The importance of clearly defining rights and responsibilities as part of the open exchange of information has received increased attention in child welfare over the past few years, particularly in the form of written service or treatment contracts. Many of the chapters in Part III emphasize the role of written service agreements in the specialist foster care scheme to assist in clearly defined placement objectives, time lines, and the mutual rights and responsibilities of each party. An important question is the extent to which the parties to the service agreement have opportunities to be involved, to participate and to openly share information and exercise choice. Do social workers dictate goals, tasks, and responsibilities? Are active efforts made to involve foster parents, youth, and birth parents in defining the terms of the placement and the goals to be achieved?

Placement Programming

Two key sets of activities central to the implementation of specialist fostering programs are the ongoing implementation, assessment, and revision of the service agreement and the provision and use by foster parents of necessary support services. Unless carefully monitored and assessed, service agreements or treatment contracts can amount to paper exercises with little substantive meaning to the actual day-to-day delivery of services to youth in care. Indeed, each significant program component needs to be carefully assessed and the information used to enhance the services delivered. Ongoing program evaluation is not a major theme in most of the papers although an exception is the evaluation system being implemented by the Human Service Associates. A dual track evaluation system has been established in that agency to conduct periodic evaluations and an ongoing monitoring system.

A question then arises about the focus of agency evaluation work, specifically the kinds of questions to be addressed in an agency evaluation system. Should the evaluation system focus on addressing follow-up questions having to do with the status of youth discharged and, if so, what criteria should be used to determine success? Alternately, should evaluation efforts place less emphasis on the youth served, and more on assessing the amount and type of services provided in the day to day life of the program and the way in which the relevant parties make key decisions about the persons served? Such a perspective on program evaluation may have the benefit of pushing program officials to think more carefully about the nature of key program elements, the interrelationships of program elements, and the bases upon which important decisions are made.

An additional key program activity in special foster care programming is the use of a variety of support services. All of the chapters in Part III emphasize the twenty-four-hour on-call availability of social workers to foster parents as well as the use of support groups. These groups amount to a web of relationships, a pattern of ties between small groups of treatment parents who meet on a regular basis and give and receive encouragement, support, and assistance. Other types of support groups are described in Chapter 10 by Emily Jean McFadden and her colleagues with regard to emancipating youth and in Chapter 18 in the context of respite services for treatment parents in the HSA program.

CONCLUSIONS

The papers in the volume establish the viability of specialist foster family care. They identify a number of matters and issues which will require further attention as this form of service develops. The material that follows provides some perspectives and principles regarding specialist foster family care, a discussion of program issues, and program approaches or descriptions. In the title of this volume we have used the term specialist foster family care, although as the following chapters illustrate, there is no agreement as to the proper title for this form of community care. Specialized foster care, family-based treatment, treatment foster care, and community care provider are all terms used by various authors.

In the concluding chapter we return to some of the ideas introduced here and note areas which may require further clarification as specialist foster family care develops. We suggest that two program approaches are emerging although these are not necessarily mutually exclusive, note implications for the role of foster parent and social worker in this type of foster family care, note the ambiguous relationship between permanency planning and specialist foster family care, suggest the importance of more systematic involvement of birth parents, and, finally, note the possibility of extending specialist foster care to other populations.

PART I:
PERSPECTIVES AND PRINCIPLES

Chapter 2

Looking Backwards, Looking Forwards

Nancy Hazel

ABSTRACT. Reviews developments in foster care over the last 15 years in England, outlines key program ingredients of the Kent project in respect to these developments and identifies several matters bearing on services for youth which need further consideration and development.

As I have been concerned with foster care singe 1950, I thought I might briefly reflect as a kind of ancient monument—looking back in order to look forward, and using my own career as a kind of mirror of the history of fostering. If I pick 1974 as the year to look back to, it is possible to see how much has changed in a relatively short time—and this is encouraging when one is tempted to think

Nancy Hazel is former Research Fellow, University of Kent School of Social Work, 27 Clifton Gardens, Canterbury, Kent CT2 8DR, United Kingdom.

17

that the same old problems are never overcome. By 1974 I had completed a study of child placement carried out with an international research group on behalf of the Council of Europe, looking at all the member countries. I followed this with a study on my own of Sweden and Belgium. Up to that time I had been an English social worker and social work teacher and had believed (more or less) what I was told by my elders and betters. At that time the wisdom of the profession was that many children were unsuitable for fostering or adoption, because they were too old, too unhealthy, inconvenient parents, and so on.

It was a period of specialized institutions when children were sent far away from their homes to institutions for younger delinquent boys, for older difficult girls, to special boarding schools for every kind of handicap, and so on. Department of Health and Social Services officials were pressing for more residential provision, and indeed foster care in England was not very successful. Research at that time tended to lay the blame either on the child, the parents, or the foster family. The contribution of the social worker or departmental policy was seldom analyzed. But I had discovered in Sweden a public system in which even adolescent drug abusers could be fostered, where the rate of fostering was very high and the use of institutions low. Belgium, on the other hand, based its child care system on residential care and relied heavily on non-state organizations. Austria, France, Germany and the Netherlands were also quite different. So it became clear to me that a country could have any kind of system; my English smugness was shattered once and for all.

This long story has several points. First, how important it is for us to be in touch and ready to learn from each other from country to country. Second, beware of false certainties. In 1974 in England, we *knew* that many children were unsuitable for fostering, that adolescents could not be fostered, that only healthy babies were suitable for adoption and so on (although of course there were exceptions in practice). Today the problem is reversed—*no* person is unsuitable for family placement, although it may not be possible to provide the family environment which would be suitable for particular people. Today the idea seems quite extraordinary that we could have defined so many children and young people as unsuitable for living in ordinary family life, and could have sent them away so far from their homes rather than trying to integrate them into their local communities and schools.

In 1974 I wanted to kill off one of these certainties—that delinquent or disturbed adolescents can only be accommodated in institutions—and that was the origin of the Kent Project. This was a five-year experimental project aiming to place the most disturbed and delinquent adolescents aged 15 to 17 in families and to publish the methods and results. It was surprisingly successful, partly because the tide of social policy was turning away. It is no longer an experiment and has been widely accepted as a model (Hazel, 1981).

The role of the social worker had been seen mainly in terms of relationships, emotional understanding, and unravelling the child's past. The Kent Project tried to shift the emphasis to objectives and tasks in the present. We relied heavily on American writing on task-centered casework (Reid & Epstein, 1972; Reid, 1978) and were encouraged by the Massachusetts experience at closing institutions for delinquents and specialized family placement schemes in Minnesota (Galaway, 1972, 1976, 1978) and Alberta (Larson, Allison, & Johnston, 1978). From these borrowed ideas, the Kent Project produced a recipe which has stood the test of time. The ingredients include the following: (1) *Egalitarianism.* Social workers, foster parents, youth and families are all equal in esteem and status. Work proceeds as a partnership. (2) *Good pay for difficult and skilled work.* The foster parents are independent fee-earning professionals. (3) *Working together in groups.* The foster parents support each other rather than depending on the social worker. (4) *Written contracts.* Based on the principle of openness, written contracts specify the overall objective and the duration of the placement, the specific tasks to be tackled, the contribution of each party to the agreement and the arrangements for termination. Since 1975 the Kent recipe has remained unchanged, although sometimes diluted.

Let us jump to the present. In England emphasis is now on closing institutions and the development of fostering—a complete reversal since 1974. At that time it would have been unthinkable for a county to experiment with working without any residential care as is the case in Warwickshire today. Foster care is changing from being a mass of undifferentiated substitute homes, were money was a dirty word (of course foster parents worked for love) to a continuum of varied careers. The continuum includes short-stay and emergency, rehabilitation, and bridging foster care; link families to support the parents of severely handicapped children; professional fostering for disturbed or delinquent older children or adolescents; and permanency which is almost the same as adoption. The first group of careers are now generally paid as skilled work, whereas money is not so much a reward for work done as a means to continue caring for an extra child in placements which offer a permanent home.

The ideology of the Kent project was egalitarianism, good pay, written contracts and working together in groups. Pay for skilled work is now generally accepted. Foster parents are still somewhat suspicious of working together in groups, but I think this is important as they are the real experts and can help each other. Opportunities for training for foster parents have developed with training and status closely linked. Unfortunately foster parents are still generally seen as people to be trained rather than as a pool of experts who can play an important part in the training of social workers. Written contracts are both widely used but also resisted. Jane Rowe has been chairing a national working party for the National Foster Care Association, trying to promote written agreements for all placements. In special fostering schemes working together in partnership and the use of written agreements is well advanced, but elsewhere social workers were often less open and foster parents often resistant to written agreements. There may still be places where foster parents are not invited to case conferences or included in reviews, but this would not now be regarded as good practice; the right of people to see their personal files is now accepted in principle even though it may be difficult to implement in practice. So there is still much to be done to achieve the goals of equality and openness in day-to-day practice.

Perhaps the greatest change has been in the status of the natural family. In the past birth parents were often excluded and not considered as equals, but there is now a new emphasis on returning children home. A government White Paper has produced recommendations which emphasize the need for a partnership between the child's parents and the local authority. There is emphasis on the importance of in-and-out patterns of care like the arrangements made to help the parents of handicapped children. Children in care now tend to be older, and it is vital to include their own family; recent research suggests that in-and-out patterns, using the same foster family, work well. But the development of this kind of fostering makes it imperative to kill off certain old ideas such as "care is to be avoided at all costs," "preventing entry to care" and so on. Care must be seen as a positive step, a safe and constructive experience – and we must make it so in reality. All this is very basic common sense on the principle that "a stitch in time saves nine." And once again work of this kind can only proceed on a basis of equal partnership and openness.

For foster parents the career which is now developing is one of partnership with the natural family in three ways: (1) Working with a family at referral to help them survive together rather than breaking up. (2) Maintenance during the child's time in care by acting as a refuge in times of stress or complementing the natural family in a variety of ways. (3) Rehabilitation by helping the child to return home.

We need to give attention to the role of foster parents in aftercare when the placement is over. The contribution of foster parents to aftercare has been immense and generally not recognized. Life is truly bleak for an adolescent who does not live at home and has no trusted adult to turn to in times of change or stress. Foster parents, even where the placement has seemed to be a failure, often remain permanent friends and helpers – but at their own expense. This needs to be changed.

I am presently promoting a small scheme to accommodate homeless 16- to 20-year olds in families. We accept both those who have been in care and those who have never entered care. The plight of adolescents who are homeless after leaving care is bad enough, but at least the social services departments are permitted under law to befriend them; the situation of those who have never been in care is even worse. If they cannot continue to live at home for various reasons – death or illness of parents or trouble with stepparents for example – they are no one's responsibility. It is very hard for them to find anywhere to live. If they are unemployed they are moved on every few weeks under the Social Security regulations. If they manage to find work they cannot usually earn enough to pay their way and are not usually eligible for a housing benefit. Without adult friends their life is impossible. The Canterbury scheme is based on a small voluntary organization which runs a youth center. It has made a good start. Referrals flood in and families, as ever, are willing to help. It is in fact a rather promising scheme; the model seems to work and it is very cheap to run.

There are a number of schemes in existence for 16- to 20-year-old young people, but most of them consist of a hostel or grouped bedsitters rather than a network of families. Young people are supposed to prefer hostels or bedsitters for independent living, and, of course, many of them do. But my experience suggests that this is not true for all youths, particularly the most lonely and deprived. Is this the same old sacred cow of "adolescents are unsuitable for family placement" all over again?

There are two main tasks for the future. (1) The development and improvement of social work and caring skills so that we offer children and their parents a better service. (2) The further extension of family placement to other groups including young homeless adults, the old, mentally ill, and handicapped people. The big question is how far families in the community can support the deviant and rejected ones, and what resources and help do they need to enable them to carry out this work?

Chapter 3

Treating Emotionally Disturbed Children and Adolescents in Foster Homes

Pamela Meadowcroft

ABSTRACT. Treatment foster care is a relatively new form of service to emotionally disturbed children and adolescents. Although there is not agreement on the term to use to define this model (e.g., therapeutic foster care, special foster care, foster family-based treatment, or individual residential treatment), all programs treating these youngsters within substitute families share certain characteristics: (1) treatment of only one or two children within the homes of carefully selected substitute families; (2) low caseloads (5 to 15); (3) frequent, treatment-oriented supervision of the treatment parents that promotes a therapeutic relationship with the child; (4) provision of treatment services that are well-documented for each child; (5) professionalizing treatment parents through intensive pre-service and in-service training, good pay, and frequent performance evaluations; (6) intensive support services to treatment parents; (7) crisis intervention services; (8) education liaison; (9) health screening and medical services; and (10) coordination of each child's system of care.

PURPOSE AND BACKGROUND

The purpose of this paper is to summarize the current status of treatment foster care for seriously emotionally disturbed children, to provide a general framework for defining what this model of care is and to demonstrate the special promise that treatment foster

Pamela Meadowcroft is Director of PRYDE: Family Based Treatment, Pressley Ridge School, 530 Marshall Avenue, Pittsburgh, PA 15214.

homes have for many children who are currently or will be institutionalized.

The deinstitutionalization movement for troubled teens began about fifteen years ago. Jerome Miller's passionate pursuit of closing training schools in Massachusetts, Pennsylvania, and elsewhere, along with the push for least restrictive settings for all handicapped children and the generally poor conditions of institutional care, created the Zeitgeist for community-based treatment. Those who promoted closing residential settings for troubled teens pointed out that the staff/youth ratio was often one-to-one. It would make better sense, be more humane, possibly even more effective, and certainly less costly, if each staff person took one child home. So the reasoning went. The Pressley Ridge Schools in Pittsburgh, Pennsylvania used this logic in 1981 in closing their residential program for 50 adolescent boys and girls and placing these children in the homes of professional foster parents. The experiences of these PRYDE families have had will be quoted throughout this paper.

Although treatment foster care is considered the least restrictive residential option for troubled youths, this does not imply that it is the least *intensive* treatment option. Restrictiveness does not have a direct relationship to treatment intensity and therefore severity of behavior problems that can be treated within a particular setting (Hawkins & Luster, 1982; Stroul & Friedman, 1986). Extremely disturbed and multiply handicapped children can be and have been served in treatment foster homes (Burge, Fabry, Conoway, & James, 1987). Whether a child can be successfully served in special foster care will be determined by the program's strengths, availability of highly skilled foster families, and community resources. Only a very small number of children must have their treatment needs met in a congregate facility. Given the proper treatment homes and resources, a large percentage of children currently in psychiatric hospitals, group homes, residential treatment centers, or detention facilities can be more successfully served in a family setting. Envision psychiatrists or psychologists making house calls to these treatment homes. Why not take the professionals to the child rather than congregating children for the convenience of the professionals? Instead of considering treatment foster care as foster care at its best, why not consider it as residential treatment at its best (family oriented, great staff to child ratio, and excellent adult and peer role models).

CURRENT STATUS OF TREATMENT FOSTER CARE

The most recent reviews of existing treatment foster care programs yield some consistent patterns. The programs tend to be quite new and small. An audience survey at the First North American Treatment Foster Care Conference (Meadowcroft, 1987) of more than 400 participants indicated that 100 programs providing special foster homes to troubled children from all regions of the United States and several from Canada were represented at the conference. Of all these programs only half had a service history of more than two years. Few programs (10 percent) existed more than 10 years ago. Nearly half of all the programs were small, serving 20 or fewer children. Only a small number, less than 10 percent, were serving more than 100 children.

A recent, national study of treatment foster care (Stroul & Goldman, in preparation) showed comparable findings. This review focused on a selection of about 35 model treatment foster care programs that were recommended by state offices of mental health as exemplars of community-based care for seriously emotionally disturbed children. Within this select sample of programs, 40 percent served fewer than 20 children and only 10 percent served more than 60. Most of the programs were private, nonprofit agencies that subcontracted for services to public child mental health or child welfare agencies. Most of the programs served older children and adolescents and all served children who were considered emotionally disturbed or behavior disordered. Few characterized the population they served as seriously violent or actively psychotic.

Although these two recent reviews of treatment foster care yield some quantitative similarities, there are great differences within states and even within circumscribed regions of the country. Within Pennsylvania over 55 programs consider their services to be special foster care for over 2,000 emotionally disturbed and medically needy (including AIDS) children (Pierce, 1987). The largest program in this state serves over 450 children and adolescents in specialized foster care homes and was developed only eight years ago.

In Allegheny County, Pennsylvania, where Pittsburgh PRYDE is located, 10 special foster care programs serve about 250 children of which 100 are placed in 75 PRYDE homes including a few seriously violent, dually diagnosed children for whom even residential care had failed. Since 1,200 youngsters require out-of-home services (i.e., foster family, group home, institutional, emergency shelter) within this county, special foster care provides 20 percent of all the bed space for these children (Allegheny County CYS, 1987; Carros & Kriksten, in preparation).

Just two years ago West Virginia had fewer than 120 children in special foster care. That figure has since doubled. West Virginia PRYDE, initiated within this period, had a population of 55 children by September, 1987 including six Intensive PRYDE youths who were the beginning of the state's efforts to return 100 children placed in expensive, out-of-state psychiatric hospitals or residential treatment centers. The seriously violent, unpredictable, and medically involved nature of these children's problems made them especially difficult to treat in any setting. Nonetheless, these youngsters are succeeding well in treatment foster homes and are true examples of the potential treatment foster care has for seriously emotionally disturbed children.

The state of Maryland, which borders Pennsylvania, has just begun to develop treatment foster care. As of mid-1987 only about 100 children of all ages were being served in special foster care. The state has identified at least an additional 200 children who need treatment foster homes with the possibility of diverting many more children from residential care and reducing lengths of stay in residential treatment centers (Goss, 1987). Treating AIDS children in special foster homes, especially infants and young children, is being developed as a preferred treatment plan to expensive hospitalization for an indefinite time.

To summarize, the rapid proliferation of treatment foster care for seriously emotionally disturbed children began within the past five years. Most programs are new and serve a small number of children and adolescents. But among these programs there is already a zealousness. Staff and treatment foster parents see the damage that years of institutional care did to many of the children in their care. They see the results that can be achieved in a normal family setting even with children most others have given up on. And they see this as their challenge.

DEFINING TREATMENT FOSTER CARE

Treatment foster care cannot be easily defined. The variations in the model and its recent and rapid growth prevent a consolidated definition of what it is or is not. Inherently the model changes to fit the very individual needs of children. Some children may have daily contact with psychiatric services or require a foster parent aide within the home because of violent behavior or the need for 24-hour, within-eyesight supervision. This flexibility is one of its greatest advantages yet also prevents easily defining the model.

Even after extensive discussions across many programs, this model of care has no consistent label. With different degrees of treatment intensity, different expectations of treatment parents, different degrees of structure within the foster homes, programs have adopted different terms to describe their models. Thus there is "therapeutic foster care," "treatment foster care," "foster family-based treatment," "special foster care" and "individual residential treatment" (*Therapeutic foster care*, 1986).

Many treatment foster care programs prefer to have no or little association with "foster care." Traditionally foster care has not served as a treatment environment but rather as a substitute family environment. The biases of this history create skepticism among professionals that seriously troubled children can be well served in such unrestrictive settings. Poor pay to foster families, no or poor quality of care often provided within foster homes, and generally poor results with the seriously troubled, older child create other reasons for distinguishing treatment foster care from traditional forms of foster care. Many treatment foster care programs have no prior experience with traditional foster care but instead have service histories grounded in residential care or psychiatric hospitalization (Snodgrass & Bryant, 1984). Thus some treatment foster care programs do not mention foster care within their program descriptions and may even be licensed as residential care rather than foster care. However, for the purpose of this paper "treatment foster care" or "special foster care" will be used to describe programs providing treatment for children with the private homes of families.

Generally treatment foster care programs fit within two broad categories (Stroul & Friedman, 1986; Trout & Meadowcroft, 1985). The first category includes programs that provide the foster parents with a modest increase over traditional foster care payments, some general training, and frequent supervision, and that rely primarily on the family environment as the main therapeutic intervention. The second category includes programs that treat the foster parent more as an employee than a volunteer, as is the case in traditional foster care. Thus foster parents in this category receive more technical training, have responsibilities for implementing treatment plans within the home and community, and are paid a stipend or salary that would be equivalent to a beginning child care worker's pay. Even among treatment foster parents there is a strong sense of departure from foster care:

> I don't consider myself a foster parent. I'm a treatment parent. That means I receive professional training, certification and ongoing supervision for working with a child who has serious problems. As a parent, I care for a troubled child in my home. As a treatment parent I am a teacher and I teach the child a variety of adaptive behaviors such as how to get along with peers, how to do school work, how to express feelings, how to fit into a family, and how to succeed within a community. I really see myself as a professional.

Even though there are variations in size and substance among treatment foster care programs within these two broad categories, all have some characteristics in common. The following ten features should be present in any program that is serving as a foster family treatment environment for troubled/troubling children (Pierce, 1987).

1. A Safe, Nurturing Family for Typically One or Two Troubled Children

The most common characteristic of all special foster care programs is the setting—within the private home of a substitute family—and the number of children placed. Each treatment family provides the child with room and board including sufficient bedroom space for the child's privacy and appropriate clothes so that the child will fit well into the family and community. Children are placed within families who can best meet the child's treatment needs as well as ethnic needs; whenever possible minority children are placed within minority families who are capable of being sensitive to this child's culture. Thus the model has the capability of being more culturally sensitive than congregate care and obviously more family centered.

Treatment foster care, unlike traditional foster family care or group home care, typically finds no more than two foster children placed per treatment home. A number of programs try to limit each treatment home to one child while there are those that, in unusual circumstances, place up to five children (often this includes at least one sibling group or an adolescent mother and child). No evidence to date indicates that treatment homes with only one foster child succeed better than those with two. But typically the programs strive for a rich staff (treatment parents included) to child ratio so the proper supervision and teaching within the home is possible.

Because treatment parents are required to participate in extensive pre-service and in-service training and to implement professionally developed treatment plans, those who become treatment parents are highly functioning, well adjusted, highly committed parents with the "right stuff." A feature of this model is its emphasis on recruiting highly skilled families.

> I was put on this earth to perform one miracle. When Terry first came to our house, we knew we were his last chance before the decision would be to send him to a psychiatric hospital. They called him psychotic. To see Terry today playing with my others kids in the backyard is that one miracle I needed to perform.

Recruitment of these families is the biggest barrier to successfully launching a treatment foster care program. Within a six-month period in Pittsburgh PRYDE, 198 potential treatment parents contacted the program. After this initial call only 53 percent requested an application. Many discovered PRYDE was not for them—the job was not foster care and the children needing help were older, troublesome teenagers. Of the 104 applications sent, only 55 percent were returned. Another round of self selection resulted from the extensive application forms. Of the 57 applications received, only 75 percent of the families were scheduled for an interview. Some families, it was clear from their applications, were inappropriate for PRYDE parenting or after further discussions chose not to be interviewed. Of those who completed the interview only 80 percent were invited to the pre-service training; only 20 completed the training; and only 12 families actually served a child. Beginning with 198 families and ending with 12—only 6 percent—means that programs needing family resources must continuously create ongoing, keen interest in the program and build-in multistage screening so that families have several opportunities to select themselves out before the program does.

As in foster care programs, treatment foster care finds that the best recruitment activities involve foster parents who are already serving a child. Over 60 percent of the PRYDE families are recruited through other PRYDE families (Hawkins, Meadowcroft, Trout, & Luster, 1985; Grealish, Hunt, Lynch, & James, 1987). Recruitment activities should therefore involve treatment parents. For example, home introduction parties in which treatment parents invite promising couples to their home to learn about the program from the professional staff have proven to be very effective in producing families who eventually serve a child. By relying on other treatment parents, however, a program must be committed to recruiting highly skilled families at the beginning of the program. Compromising on parent quality to merely build-up the number of families available will eventually create a weak pool of treatment families.

Many treatment foster care programs find that the population of treatment foster parents differ from traditional foster parents. Only about 10 percent of the treatment parents in PRYDE had prior experience as foster parents. Families to target include those who are eager to have a career or professional training in working with seriously troubled children. Emphasizing the professional aspects and expectations of the job as well as the difference it can make in a child's life will attract promising couples. Most treatment foster care programs also find that they cannot limit their recruitment to couples in which only one works outside the home. Although this is desirable, it is more important to find couples who have flexible work schedules and who demonstrate the skills and commitment necessary to implementing a prescribed treatment plan.

There is no reason to believe that treatment families are a scarce resource. The difficulties programs have in recruiting families result more from failing to devote sufficient energies to recruitment activities, failing to target the appropriate population and/or failing to provide sufficient pay to attract parents interested in the professional aspects of treatment parenting than to a lack of interest within the community to help children. Within a two-year period the West Virginia PRYDE program had 55 youngsters placed in 40 homes and had successfully served an additional 20 children. The families are there, even in rural settings, for the continued development and expansion of treatment foster care services.

2. Low Caseloads

The next most common characteristic of treatment foster care is a necessary low child to staff ratio. Case management staff, or parent supervisors, typically carry a caseload of no more than 15 children. The most typical caseload is 10 although several programs report caseloads as low as 5 or 7. Programs having caseloads this small typically require parent supervisors to work with the child's natural family, assist with recruitment and other training activities, do extensive liaison work with external resources (e.g., schools), and, in some cases, provide follow-up services when the child is discharged home.

3. Frequent Treatment-Oriented Supervision

Low caseloads allow the parent supervisors to visit the treatment homes once a week or more often if necessary, especially during initial placement and during crises. Home supervision meetings can require up to three hours of interaction time to review the week's events, conduct in-home training of the treatment parents, provide a supportive ear to the family, and meet the child, if necessary.

The focus of supervision meetings is on facilitating a therapeutic relationship between the child and treatment parents. Therefore, the parent supervisor will try to provide the foster parents with the skills they need to achieve the desired behavior change or be able to successfully conduct in-home talk sessions with the child. This therapeutic relationship can be seen from the words of one PRYDE teenager:

> You know, at first I had a real hard time learning new ways. I though that if I learned how to interact 'appropriately' that I wouldn't fit in any more. But now I know I can talk street talk and be cool when I want. I used to act so ignorant to people. I though that was the way to be cool. Now I can get along better with more kinds of people. I finally figured out that what my PRYDE parents were teaching me was just adding to who I am, so I can make it and be successful. It doesn't take anything away from who I am.

4. Provision of Treatment Services

Treatment services vary widely across treatment foster care and even within each program depending on the individual needs of the youngsters. However, all treatment foster care programs assess each child's need for different services, provide counseling either through program staff or external agency resources and emphasize teaching by the treatment parents of age appropriate behaviors in the home, community, and schools.

Children within these programs have significant mental health and in some instances, physical health (e.g., AIDS, cerebral palsy, deafness, blindness) problems that require well planned and monitored services. The children typically have had prior multiple placements, are most often older children or adolescents, had their first mental health or child welfare contact at the age of nine, have special education needs, are frequently aggressive either with peers, adults or both and have histories involving other status offenses or antisocial behavior such as running away, truancy, vandalism, lying, or sexual misconduct (Hawkins et al., 1985; Trout & Meadowcroft, 1985; Stroul & Goldman, in preparation). The children come from families having long histories of family stressors including poverty, marital discord, drug/alcohol abuse, mental illness, and child abuse/neglect.

My wife and I have been PRYDE parents for five years and have worked with several kids. Our first PRYDE son, Ray, was the most undersocialized person we had ever met. Ray didn't have many conversation skills, and if he did talk it was to perseverate on violence. He talked more to himself than to other people, often having conversations with himself in different voices. He had been badly burned in a house fire when he was two and has spent most of his time hiding from people, both physically and emotionally. He would threaten me or become aggressive if he made the slightest mistake. He wanted to be perfect. (Goss, 1986)

To ensure that these very troubled children receive the various services they need while in a treatment home requires close monitoring of each case. Within PRYDE, for example, at entry each child has a written treatment plan developed much like an individualized educational program (IEP). The child, his/her treatment parents, natural parents, the treatment parent supervisor, and local county caseworker all develop and agree on a written set of general goals to be achieved while the child is in PRYDE. From this signed document a set of very specific daily objectives is written that determine what the child and treatment parents must accomplish each day. Although every child's plan differs because each enters with different problems, common objectives include "follows PRYDE parent instruction without complaining" or "reports whereabouts when not at home" or "shares feelings about the day in a calm voice" or "says something positive about himself." The treatment parents record completion of each objective on a daily form and engage the child in a "teaching episode." A teaching episode may include having the child practice the skill more completely or just letting the child know how much the treatment parents appreciate the child's efforts. Completion of the objectives determines the child's privileges and thus the child is motivated to learn and discover, perhaps for the first time, that his/her behavior has consistent results. These daily records, along with a daily log completed by treatment parents that reviews critical events of the day and the child's activities of the day, provide detailed information for revising the treatment plan, evaluating the child's progress, and evaluating the treatment parents' quality of care. Monitoring treatment goals, ensuring a positive, family focus on them, and having consistent consequences for achieving them are all aspects of accountable treatment in treatment foster care (Hawkins & Meadowcroft, 1984; Fabry, Meadowcroft, Frost, Hawkins, & Conoway, 1987).

Traditional counseling, regular talk sessions with a professional therapist or counselor, has a role in most treatment foster care programs. However, the role of the counselor as the change agent needs to be modified since that is often the responsibility of the treatment parents. In such cases the therapist functions as a clinical consultant to the treatment team which would include the treatment parents and their supervisor. The clinician's role is one of assessing the child's difficulties and advising the treatment team on ways to help the child within the treatment home and community. As a consultant to the team, rather than the child's therapist, the clinician's relationship with the child would not undermine that which the treatment parents have, or are trying to establish.

5. Professionalizing Treatment Parents

Treatment foster care regards treatment parents as extensions of their professional staff. The foster parents are well paid and receive regular evaluations that in some instances may determine pay increases. A useful guideline for establishing pay for treatment parents is to consider doubling whatever the local foster parent rate is. The training requirements, in-home treatment plan, and intensive supervision of treatment parents make this a job requiring compensation beyond the cost of the child's daily care. In programs where the pay is only slightly above regular foster care payments, parent recruitment is more difficult, expectations of the treatment parents are often lower, and more severe youngsters cannot be served.

6. Support Services for Treatment Families

Our PRYDE supervisor worked so closely with us, planning interventions with Mary. At times we had to meet or talk several times a day because Mary was an extremely difficult child. We'd develop an intervention and then evaluate to decide if we needed to try another approach. It is a lot of work, but Mary is getting along much better with her peers, is participating in more group activities, and she is learning, sometimes painfully, what it means to have friends. Having been terribly abused she was a completely nonsocial child when she entered our PRYDE home. Mary can now play simple board games with our other children. She recently joined a softball team with one of our kids and even helps with her paper route. Mary is just now beginning to talk a little about the years of abuse she suffered in her parents' home. This is an extremely important area that must be dealt with if Mary is to begin to leave the pain, fear, and guilt behind her and make her own life. Finally, Mary's small successes have begun to convince her of her own worth as a person. (Reitz, 1987)

Skeptics of this model claim that seriously emotionally disturbed children cannot receive sufficiently intense treatment by nonprofessionals, the treatment parents. Yet the data to date suggest that these skeptics are wrong. Of the 83 youngsters discharged from PRYDE through February, 1985, over 70 percent successfully completed enough of their goals that they were able to be placed in lesser restrictive settings (home, foster care, adoption, or independent living) (Trout, 1985). In a follow-up study conducted during 1986 to 44 youngsters discharged one or two years earlier, 73 percent of the children were living in settings less restrictive than PRYDE and 71 percent had had no known police contacts or other antisocial episodes (Kriegish, Richardson, Lichtenfels, Lilley, Fabry, & Hawkins, 1986). These successes were achieved even though the median length of stay, 12 months, did not exceed that for more restrictive (and more costly) residential treatment centers. To the skeptics we need to point out that mental health professionals may also be as successful as treatment parents if they live with these children 24 hours a day, seven days a week.

Treatment parents' success with seriously emotionally disturbed foster children is due in large part to the support they receive from the program's professional staff. The intensity and variety of support services to treatment families is another hallmark of treatment foster care (Meadowcroft & Grealish, 1985). These supports most often include:

(a) A multi-session pre-service training (at least four, two-hour sessions) and frequent in-service training workshops (at least four, two-hour sessions a year although eight would be more ideal) that require the attendance of all treatment parents. Couples who may have no professional experience in child care need to learn to perform well a set of useful therapeutic skills as well as learn about issues regarding foster care, special education, child development, childhood psychopathology, and specific strategies for dealing with problems typical to this population of children.

(b) Respite care for the treatment parents. Treatment foster care programs provide respite in a variety of ways. Some hire and train separate respite workers who provide services in the treatment parents' home. Others recruit and train treatment parents who do only respite work within their homes. Active treatment parents may provide respite to each other in a reciprocal arrangement. Still other programs provide respite through a combination of all of these. Respite care must be a feature of this model. It helps prevent parent burnout and provides the program with another familiar family for the child if he or she must be moved to another treatment home.

(c) 24-hour on-call service which is staffed by the program's professional workers. This service functions as an emergency linkage for the treatment parents to staff. Staff must be available to respond within minutes of the call either through problem solving on the phone, going to the treatment home to assist the family, or bringing together a crisis intervention team that can be at the home within a short period of time. Responding to treatment parents' calls requires a staffing pattern that allows for availability of staff at all hours of the night, weekends, and holidays. Staff may need to carry beepers through which they can be reached while not at home or office.

(d) Frequent, treatment-oriented, supportive supervision. One aspect of this feature not described earlier is the supportive quality of the supervision. The main responsibility of parent supervisors is to ensure that the treatment parents have skills they need to help the child and that they do not become overly stressed, i.e., to take care of the treatment parents so they can provide high quality care for the child. Staff are not directly responsible for the well-being of the child—only through supervising the treatment parents. Therefore, treatment parents need to be able to talk freely to their supervisor, to feel well-liked and respected for the tough job they are doing, to feel empowered by the program staff members' visit to their home, and ultimately to feel as though this professional is a colleague and friend. In this context the treatment parents will discuss their mistakes more freely and the program will be able to prevent many of the reoccurring abuses so common in traditional foster care. Since PRYDE's inception in 1981 with over 250 children served, it has not had a single case of treatment parent abuse because of good parent selection, training, and, most importantly, staff support.

(e) Support groups for treatment parents. Treatment parents often learn best from other treatment parents and feel part of a larger group when they have frequent opportunities to meet. Treatment parents' meetings may occur along with the in-service training workshops. Parents have the chance to form networks, to share successes, and encourage those who may be experiencing some failures. Some programs design networks of treatment families, or clusters, of five to six families that meet as often as once a week, share respite care within the group, and get to know each child being served by each family (Gideon, 1986). Other programs allow informal networks to develop through the program workshops by providing parents with small group discussion formats and everyone's phone numbers.

(f) Other supports that programs have used include special letters or certificates of recognition for noteworthy accomplishments of the parents, bonuses or a special dinner for extra intervention work during a particularly troublesome period with the child, participation of the parents in program development (e.g., parent advisory board, parent training assistants, parent recruitment assistants), and even hiring treatment parents for different program jobs (e.g., as parent supervisors themselves).

7. Crisis Intervention Services

Crises will happen in the homes, community or schools. If a program experiences no serious acting-out, runaways, or other serious antisocial behavior, then it is not serving the more troublesome child for whom treatment foster care is designed. Yet a program should not be buffeted from one crisis to another. Taking appropriate prevention measures (e.g., high levels of structure within the home and intensive supervision of the child) helps minimize the frequency and severity of these events (Fabry & James, 1985). When the events occur, the program's response determines the immediate outcome for the child and family and the longer-term maintenance of treatment parents. As described in the section on 24-hour on-call service, being able to respond within minutes to a problem within the home, community or school is the first priority.

The second component of crisis intervention is forming crisis intervention teams. Crisis teams prevent one staff member from having to manage an episode of aggression or injury to the child and/or family by themselves. A crisis team may need to include psychiatric/psychological professionals as well as staff most familiar with the child and family. Treatment foster care programs must also have backup placement options for each child. An event may occur which requires removing the child from his or her treatment home (e.g., abusing a younger child in the home, the treatment family insisting on removal for a cooling-off period, etc.). Backup placements may include (1) other treatment homes; (2) a program-operated home that is staffed with professionals or a specially skillful couple, who are particularly prepared to work with youngsters in crisis; (3) a diagnostic unit operated by the program for short-term assessment and crisis resolution; (4) arrangements with local psychiatric hospitals, other mental health facilities, or detention facilities for short-term stays with the goal of returning the child to the treatment home after the crisis has been resolved.

8. Education Services

A majority of the children in treatment foster care have special education needs. Treatment foster care programs need to assess the child's educational needs and then ensure that they are provided within the community in which the child is placed. In rural programs, appropriate educational services are often difficult to find. A child may be adjusting well in the treatment home and community but be at risk for residential placement because of serious acting out within the school. These situations require strong, positive advocacy by the treatment parents and staff either to have the services created within that community, find the services within the nearest community and be prepared to provide the child with transportation, or create the services within the program. Even if appropriate education services exist, the treatment parents and staff must closely monitor the child's adjustment within that setting to prevent small problems from ending in a crisis. Education liaison is a critical service linkage within treatment foster care.

9. Health Screening and Medical Services

All children within treatment foster homes need to have regular health screenings and follow-up care. This responsibility typically rests with the treatment parents but must be well monitored by staff. Arrangements with health screening services or hospitals can improve the consistent management of this program aspect.

Children with serious medical needs can be well served within a treatment foster home. Because of the flexibility of the model, emotionally disturbed children who are also physically handicapped or are medically needy in some way can be accommodated in treatment homes. Special medical services for individual children can be more finely tuned by the treatment parents' focus on one child's needs. Medical foster care, not the focus of this paper but an interesting evolution of the model, provides a good home environment to a child who would otherwise be hospitalized for an extended time. The child's physical well-being is assured by recruiting nurses to serve as the treatment parents, paying them a salary comparable to that which they would receive through hospital employment, providing the home with all the necessary medical equipment, all for a fraction of hospital costs.

Families often are able to get the individual services a child needs more easily than larger, inherently impersonal residential programs. And a child has a family helping him or her through the medical experience.

> The night before our PRYDE child went into the hospital for one of three, 15-hour surgical procedures to reconstruct his horribly scarred face, he asked, "Will I be OK when they cut my face off?" We were horrified but realized that he was right. The team of surgeons who were donating much of their

services to this cause, were going to replace nearly all of the skin on his face from skin they "grew" on his arms—the one place where there was unscarred, soft skin left. This whole experience was intense and the beginning of physical affection for him. He was in intensive care and tubes coming out of every part of his body. His head was literally as big as a basketball but it was the neatest bit of stitchery imaginable. When I walked into the room, he put out his hand so I could hold it. He couldn't see anything because of the swelling but he could feel the drainage and the swelling. He tried to reassure us by saying, "It's good. It has to drain. I can take it." There weren't many places to touch him because they had to take an artery from his leg to put in his face and skin from his arms. We could only touch his hands and feet. But throughout the surgery experience, there was an important message that he really got—people care about him! (Goss, 1986)

10. Coordination of Services
or Ensuring System Linkages

Because the children served in treatment foster homes have multiple problems, successfully maintaining them in a family requires coordination of many different services. Some of these services have already been described: mental health, education, and health. Others that treatment parents and staff need to address include vocational services (e.g., career education, job survival training, work experience, job finding or sheltered employment); recreation within the community (after school, during summer months, special recreation projects for emotionally disturbed, handicapped children); social services (visitation with natural family, adoption, court reviews); and operational or support services (transportation, advocacy, legal services, support groups, and case management) (Stroul & Friedman, 1986).

But development of these services either within the program or external to it within the community, does not ensure that each child will receive what he or she needs in a consistent fashion. The types of services each child may need cut across funding streams and different organizations that traditionally have not worked well together (Stroul & Friedman, 1986). A child may be in a treatment home, attend a day treatment program for his/her education/mental health needs, be working at McDonalds, and attend group meetings for victims of sex abuse. To ensure that the child receives and follows through on the appropriate services when or she needs them and that the services change when needed, requires the treatment foster program to be organized in such a fashion to permit good, complete case management, frequent reviews of the child's progress, and close coordination with child welfare or child mental health.

SUMMARY

Within the past few years we have seen the development of many programs that have features of treatment foster care. Many children who would have otherwise been institutionalized or would have remained in institutional programs for long periods of time, have been successfully served in family settings. But the growth of this model is not without problems.

To ensure that treatment foster care continues to develop as an alternative to residential care, providers of this service need to contribute actively to revolutionizing children's mental health care. The historic biases within child welfare and mental health are against treating children with serious mental health or physical health needs within family settings. Professionals and policy makers continue to confuse treatment capability and intensity with the location of the service; i.e., institutional settings are considered inherently more treatment-intensive than a family setting (U.S. Congress, Office of Technology Assessment 1986).

Yet treatment technologies for seriously emotionally disturbed children exist that are easily transferable to home settings and implementable by parents (Braukmann, Fixsen, Kirigin, Phillips, Phillips, & Wolf, 1975; Hawkins, et al., 1985; Kirigin, Braukmann, Atwater, & Wolf, 1982; O'Dell, 1974; Phillips, Phillips, Fixsen, & Wolf, 1974). To redress this child mental health bias, providers of treatment foster care must be wiling to serve only those children who cannot be served in traditional foster care. They must be ready to demonstrate through adequate assessment of the children's needs and continued maintenance of program data that in fact their population of children is the neediest. They need to include all of the features described above so as to be distinct from traditional foster care, to demonstrate treatment within the foster home setting, and be able to serve more successfully a difficult population of children.

Finally, treatment foster care needs to be willing to take risks and take extraordinary steps in protecting the children, treatment parents, and the community when placing children at risk. If treatment foster care embraces these challenges, then we will see many more children having opportunities for positive family living.

The special promise of treatment foster care for children who would otherwise be institutionalized is the family-connectedness it gives to children. Once a child lives with a family for several months, he/she has a family to turn to for life. Even when, or if, the child is able to successfully return home, he/she has a treatment family as an extension of the biological family. The most successful cases of treatment foster care result in a strengthening of the child's own family through the changes the child has achieved, the changes achieved within the child's own family through program services, and the continued connection to a highly functioning family. When return home is not possible, the treatment home can provide a longer term placement, can be a potential adoptive home, or a good family to whom the young adult returns for holidays, visits, or advice on jobs, friends, or problems.

The promise treatment foster care holds is best said in a letter from a PRYDE parent. Her PRYDE son had been institutionalized for five years before entering a treatment home. His case records considered him to be an extremely antisocial child who was potentially a danger to himself and others. He was withdrawn, uncommunicative, dour, unpleasant, constantly complaining and critical of others. He was verbally and physically aggressive. The institution from which he came felt that he could make no more progress in their facility. Something else had to be tried. They predicted that he would not adjust in a PRYDE home and within six months would be in another, even more restrictive residential setting. Three years later he graduated successfully from a mainstreamed high school classroom and from PRYDE. His PRYDE mother wrote:

The day dawned the same as it always has but why on this particular day did I wake up with such mixed feelings. A little excited, proud and yet so sad and scared. The prayer that formed on my lips was, Oh God, did I really do enough? Did I do all I could have done for him. This was the day that the judge said my PRYDE child was to be on his own. He had reached 18 years of age.

Why was this day to be so different? A day is nothing more than 24 hours, a mark on the calendar, an interval of light between two successive nights. I certainly felt no different. If anything I loved him more. I had watched this scared boy of 15 walk into our home trying to act so bad yet so scared. I didn't know when it was or where it was that I realized I loved this child. It was upon me one day. We had put so much time, love, and effort into this boy that he had become a part of us that we never knew could exist.

So I say to my PRYDE child, thank you for letting us become a part of your life, thank you for allowing us to love you and help you shape your life. We hung in there together and no matter what any judge decrees that this day, this mark on the calendar, cannot erase what we have learned and lived together. I'm so proud of you. I know as I see this young man walk in the door we have both made it home.

Chapter 4

Principles and Theory of Adolescent Foster Care: A Reconsideration Following Twelve Years Practice of the Kent Family Placement Service

Peter M. Smith

ABSTRACT. Central program principles of the Kent Family Placement Service are identified and related to developments in contemporary British child care. Four areas of development in the Kent
Program are described—evaluation, client population, matching,
role of natural families—before turning to a discussion of the theoretical basis for special foster care for adolescents.

VALUE OF THEORY

Thinking about this paper has been a valuable exercise, coming
just at the end of my five-year association as a social worker with
the Kent Family Placement Service (KFPS). Having thought about
and practiced family placement, this paper presents a welcome opportunity to concentrate on theories and principles relevant to everyday practice. I want to follow the flow chart as seen in Diagram
1. This postulates theory as the origin from which principles are de-

Peter M. Smith is Development Officer (Policy & Practice), National Children's Bureau, 8 Wakley Street, London ECIV 7QE United Kingdom. The views
expressed in this chapter are those of the author and do not necessarily reflect
views of the National Children's Bureau, London.

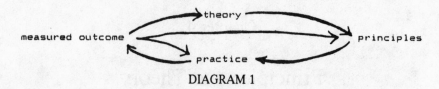

DIAGRAM 1

rived. Practice is based on principles. The outcome of practice is measured, and the results of evaluating outcome are relayed back, modifying practice, principles and theory in light of experience.

KFPS is a very pragmatic program and does not subscribe to one particular school of therapeutic thinking, because evidence of the success of one approach over another is equivocal, and because of the absolute impossibility of getting as strong-minded and varied a group as our eighty-plus families to respond to young people with a united therapeutic approach. However, to have no theory is to have no framework, no way of organizing thoughts, and no reasons for particular behavior toward young people in care, and therefore likely to leave them vulnerable to haphazard treatment which could be the result of impulse, prejudice or other purely emotional reaction. Theory is important because it underpins and guides action.

PRINCIPLES OF THE MODEL

Because the principles have changed little and have already been described by Nancy Hazel in this book and elsewhere (Hazel, 1981), this restatement will be brief.

- *Normalization*. Young people should be treated as normally as possible and with minimum stigma resulting from being in care.
- *Localization*. Young people should be allowed to live as close to home as possible in recognition of the fact that to teenagers their home town is an important aspect of their identity. This principle is modified for some young people in view of the evaluation of placement outcomes which shows that placements of teenagers deliberately away from home weakens peer group influence.

- *Participation*. Decisions about young people in care must be made with every opportunity for young people and their families to have a say.
- *Voluntarism*. A young person cannot and should not be fostered if he or she has no commitment to be with a particular family. It is acknowledged that young people would generally prefer to be somewhere else, that is with their own family, but a reluctant agreement at least to the fact of being placed with a family is essential.
- *Egalitarianism*. Lay people in their own homes can be as effective and often more effective in helping young people than highly specialized and professional residential units. As the status of foster parents has increased, the status of other workers with the young people has correspondingly decreased. The practice and results of KFPS have debunked and demystified some of the more curious aspects of psychiatric care. There have been many examples where the psychiatric symptoms of young people referred to KFPS from hospital care have spontaneously abated from the outset of the placement.

While the principles were valid in themselves, they also arose, as did the Kent Family Placement Project, as a reaction to the expansion of residential care. The Project was established to demonstrate that specialist foster care could be at least as effective as residential care. Therefore there was a crusading element to the Project which has died away. KFPS does not have the same point to prove and it is generally accepted that KFPS is the placement of choice.

The principle of normalization derives from theories of social deviance and labelling. These theories underpinned the establishment of the Kent Family Placement Project and still exercise an important influence on practice. The behavior of individuals in workplaces or in institutions is determined more than anything else by their reference group, that is their peers, friends, workmates, or fellow inmates. When an individual works or lives with a group having a particular view of the world, one's ideas will generally be overwhelmed by the values and standards of the group. This is in part true for mature adults at work, and far more true for young people in a total institution where they eat, work, learn, sleep and play. This can be illustrated from two sources, one American which dates back to the 60s and the other English, and even older.

The American sociologist Howard Polsky lived for eight months in an innovative and avowedly therapeutic home for wayward youth run on a cottage system. His book *Cottage Six* (1962) refers to the cottage for the bad lads. Polsky concluded that the social system of Cottage Six was the dominant force on the boys' lives, and this system, dominated by the boys' pecking order, undermined attempts at individual therapy. The removal of key boys from the group made no difference at all, other boys simply moved into the vacant places.

Polsky argued that the cottage organization entraps the boys in a network of social exchange from which it is difficult to escape. The tough guy, the scapegoat, the con-man and his victim all form an intense interdependent group, based not only on the cultural heritage of the cottage, but also on the boys' psychopathology. This whole set-up is implicitly supported by the staff who cooperate with the boys' organization of the cottage. So the aggressive and perhaps most ruthless member of the group will hold power, the devious will become more devious to survive and the socially inadequate learn to live at the bottom of the pile. Not only is the problem behavior of the youngsters compounded, but also the boys' image of themselves is confirmed: the winner, the con-man and the loser.

My older illustration of the power of the subgroup to determine the behavior of youngsters follows:

> The young boy and his companions suffered the tortures of slow starvation for three months: at last they got so voracious and wild with hunger, that one boy, who was tall for his age, and hadn't been used to that sort of thing (for his father had kept a small cookshop), hinted darkly to his companions, that unless he had another basin of gruel per diem, he was afraid he might some night happen to eat the boy who slept next to him, who happened to be a weakly youth of tender age. He had a wild, hungry eye; and they implicitly believed him. A council was held; lots were cast who should walk up to the master after supper that evening, and ask for more; and it fell to Oliver Twist (Dickens, 1838).

Mr. Bumble the workhouse keeper saw Oliver's behavior as evidence of moral depravity whereas Professor Polsky and others see it as a function of a deviant subculture. Literature provides many examples of the hazards of peer influence, especially in institutions (Brendan Behan, 1958). Parents know also that teenage behavior is susceptible to influence of peers. Recent research conducted at the University of Sheffield into consumer views of care illustrates how angry and disillusioned parents can be. After their teenagers had been taken into care for committing offences and being beyond control, their behavior deteriorated, largely, in the parents' view, because of the company they were keeping. Group care reinforces the socially deviant and individual community care has the chance of reinforcing the socially positive. All of us involved in fostering know this and it needs no further emphasis, save to acknowledge that the avoidance of situations which promote labeling and social deviance is the cornerstone of theory on which KFPS is based.

BASICS OF THE MODEL

In preparation for a conference in 1985 to celebrate ten years of existence, the KFPS staff group agreed that the following were the essential components of the Kent model (Kent Family Placement Service, 1985).

1. Contracts/Written Agreements. Although there is disagreement over which word to use, there is widespread agreement about the importance and the content of contracts. They must include a statement of the overall aim, the specific objectives, the schedule for review, and the nature of contact with natural family.
2. Increase status of foster parents. This is in recognition of the difficulty of their job and the need for care, control, and authority to be united to cope with teenage behavior.
3. Payment of fees. Fees have been important to recruit and retain good foster parents, and have also underlined the concept of fostering as work, helping remove naive notions of love and rescue as adequate remedies for troubled teenagers.

4. Groups. These are indispensable especially at the beginning of a fostering career to provide support and to develop expertise.

When these four essential components were presented to the 1985 conference, the foster parents demanded an addition:

5. Support Worker. His or her functions are to provide support and advice to families, to be available by phone at all times, and to get to know the families well enough to be able to make good "matches" between the needs of young people and the abilities of foster families.

The basic Kent model is very much intact; it has withstood the test of time, and according to the National (England) Foster Care Association, has been copied over seventy times in Great Britain. For the model to have survived and multiplied in this way means it is a good one. It has been a successful and influential innovation in British child care practice.

Due to the durability of the model, developments in KFPS represent changes in emphasis rather than radical departures. Subsequent research, government policy initiatives and child care trends have developed in the same direction as the Project. This is not to suggest that these developments were a result of the Project, rather that they confirm the trends illustrated.

DEVELOPMENTS IN CONTEMPORARY BRITISH CHILD CARE

Both sides of the Atlantic have seen a change in popularity of different therapies. There has been a movement from individual psychodynamically-oriented therapy towards systemic therapies which emphasize the influence of the environment. The increasing application of family therapy enables many parents to reduce emotional distress and disturbed behavior in their children by changing ways they themselves behaved. It was but a small logical step from observing that families could effectively help their own children to concluding that substitute families could be equally successful. If a child's or young person's disturbance was a result of family dynamics, then logically if a change of family dynamics could not be achieved, a change of family with a set of dynamics specifically chosen with a particular child's needs in mind could be the most effective form of treatment. Family therapy and specialist foster care are conceptually complementary.

The modern psychotherapies emphasize that clients take responsibility for changing their lives, that the therapist provides the context but the clients must provide the change. The trend is away from the mystique and omnipotence of the expert, usually medical, towards a more pragmatic and open approach to problem solving.

As well as the change in theory about how to create positive change in distressed youth, there have been modifications based on empirical testing of John Bowlby's theories of maternal deprivation. As Bowlby's theory of the primacy of the baby's attachment to the mother filtered down into social work practice, it became etched in stone. If children had suffered maternal deprivation, or maternal separation, these were grave, almost irredeemable events. The quality of care before, during, and after the separation was ignored, and Dads didn't get a mention. Simplified Bowlbyism became articles of faith. But like many certainties, they were false. The success of providing family care to those who have suffered maternal privation is now well documented in this country and the United States. Although there are higher risks with the adoption of multiply handicapped children, family care has demonstrated a resilience, effectiveness and ability to compensate for past disadvantage to a degree which would have been inconceivable twenty years ago. Thus the trend towards seeing remedies for troubled children within families was not the exclusive preserve of special foster care, but shared by trends in adoption and family therapy.

Turning attention now from a broader perspective of family care to the KFPS principles and methods, there are four interlinked concepts which were espoused by KFPS and whose absence have been lamented by recent research and reports into child care. These concepts, which have run the risk of becoming catch-phrases, are:

1. written agreements,
2. partnership with parents,
3. planning for children in care,
4. participation in decision making.

It is perhaps not immodest to suggest that the Kent Project was influential in promoting the use of written agreements in foster care. The origin of the idea is impossible to discern precisely, but the idea has certainly grown. The Social Services Select Committee of the House of Parliament (House of Commons, 1984) recommended that consideration be given to all placements being governed by written agreements. Cooper (1985) investigated the events surrounding the tragic death of Jasmine Beckford who was returned to her parents against the wishes of the foster parents and was later killed by her stepfather. As an eminent lawyer, Blom Cooper was profoundly puzzled about how placements could be effective and planned without written agreements. The contract idea still persists in the government White Paper and could be incorporated into draft legislation, which hopefully will be in the government's legislative program for Parliament in 1988/89.

Relationships between parents and foster parents and social workers can be difficult and there are hurt feelings and raw emotions that need to be addressed, but are all too often avoided. The study by J. Vernon and D. Fruin (1985) of decision making regarding children in care reported that social workers left the arranging of parental visits to foster parents, who, in turn, did not feel it was their job to do. No wonder parents of children feel pushed aside and disillusioned. Jane Rowe et al., (1984) found that in a twelve-month period social workers had only been in touch with one third of the primary parents in her sample of children in long-term foster care. The study by Millham, Bullock, Hosie, and Haak (1986) provides further evidence of dwindling links between children in care and their families. There are of course a tiny minority of parents who, for the sake of the children, should be denied access. But the decision to deny access should be made through due court process, not by administrative default.

Such shortcomings, which are persistent findings of the child care system, should not occur in a properly working family placement service. A written contract would make clear the roles, frequency of visiting, and the date of the next review. The increased status of foster parents would enable them to bring any drift away from agreements to the notice of the social workers. Through persistent obstreperousness, if nothing else, foster parents have to ensure the best service for their foster agreements. If the social worker does not have the time to contact parents, foster parents do. This is true of other aspects of the plan for the young person. It is no use for foster parents to complain about the lack of social work activity to carry out the agreed plan. Social workers have large case loads and their own priorities, whereas foster families have the interests of just one or two young people at heart and can campaign, advocate, and act on their behalf as effectively as most social workers.

It is staggering and disappointing that so many young people in care still do not attend their own reviews. Within KFPS it is accepted as obvious that all teenagers attend their contract meeting and review. In other programs there are many exceptions to this practice. It is not usual for teenagers to have any choice about placement. At the best of times choices are limited, and occasionally the social service authority can be used to make a decision for a confused younger teenager but the general principle of participation in decision making must stand.

DEVELOPMENTS IN KFPS

There have been developments in four areas:

1. evaluation,
2. changing client population,
3. the factor of emotional closeness or distance in match-making,
4. involvement of natural families.

The KFPS client group is still about 55 percent boys and 45 percent girls. However, what was seen as the typical KFPS placement — male, fifteen years of age, beyond control, truanting and heading sooner rather than later for a custodial sentence — represents a far smaller percentage of referrals than five or seven years ago. In many ways, such youngsters were better put together, more psychologically intact, than many of the teenagers currently referred. This change has come about largely because of the growth in alternative disposals in court which allow young people to remain at home with their families. Some foster parents and family placement workers regret the demise of the likeable or not so likeable rogue. Certainly last year when a "straightforward delinquent" came up for allocation at a staff meeting, there was a rush to offer suitable families.

A second difference is that the length of time children have spent in care has decreased. There are fewer referrals of young people who have been in the care system for five, seven or ten years as the social services department policy aims to avoid children growing up in care. Permanence planning is beginning to have an impact. Therefore, as a general statement, young people referred now are less likely to have long records of offending and more likely to be in greater emotional upheaval and show greater signs of emotional disturbance. This year has seen a steep rise in referrals of victims of sexual abuse.

The third area of development is the emotional dimension of the match-making, deciding which teenager is introduced to which family. This dimension seeks to match the emotional needs of the teenager and the emotional style of the foster family, and I have attempted to give it increasing attention over the years. The following questions are posed. "Is the young person's ability to give of himself or herself compatible with the family's expectations and needs which they hope will be met through fostering?" "Is there a fit between the young person's willingness to be cherished, cared for, loved, and the foster family's emotional style?" These may sound odd as questions for professional fostering, but different families give and expect returns to different degrees. I have come to think that matching the degree a family wants to give and express emotionally and the degree to which a teenager responds to this giving is the most crucial factor in determining whether the placement will be successful. I would argue that it overrides more obvious factors like social class, geography, interests, and age of own children. This emotional factor, however, is more difficult to measure and more difficult to describe.

A lad named Charlie illustrates this point. He had an economically and socially deprived background and came into care at twelve because of being beyond control and neglected. He spent the next four years in residential care despite expressing a wish to be fostered. The Social Services Department contrived to lose his parents which was quite clearly a consequence of moral judgements by his social workers about the standard of care which Charlie had suffered. Losing his family was not a reflection of his emotional needs. Even though he was sixteen, street-wise, competent to survive on long runaways and was against most of what society approved, he was desperate to be fostered. He experimented with drugs, loved rock music and styled himself after hippies.

I placed him in a very middle class family, regular Churchgoers who come across as quite proper in a very English sort of way. The foster mother tries very hard, too hard, and is not very able to distance herself emotionally from her work. Despite a bad match socially and culturally, I thought the emotional needs might mesh. Charlie has rediscovered his family with the help and support of the foster parents, is glad to have done so, but knows that they don't have a lot to offer him.

The present position is that Charlie moans to social workers and friends about his foster mother nagging him, bothering him and fussing over him, but goes out of his way to go to the foster home for lunch from work to get another dose of nagging, fussing and caring. Charlie is now eighteen. It is too early to be sure but probably the relationship between him and his foster parents will continue in an erratic way for years and years, because of the emotional congruence in an otherwise unlikely match.

This matching of emotional needs is made very easy in many experienced families because they have developed a range of emotional distances which they offer to the teenagers, depending on their age, ties with their own families, and state of the placement. They are capable of accepting into the bosom of their families those youngsters who are unable to rebuild or repair their relationships with their own families, or of retaining a professional, more distant, more matter-of-fact relationship with those teenagers on the point of returning home or moving into independence. This flexibility and range of skill on the part of foster families makes the match-maker's job very easy or almost redundant.

The fourth most crucial development has been increased acknowledgement of the importance of the teenager's own families. In 1979, fourteen of the seventy-eight teenagers followed up were at home, whereas now well over one third of those teenagers who do not break down in placement go back to their own families. From the KFPS placement outcome evaluations, it was clear that the factor most closely associated with positive outcome was the parents' attitude to the contract. Therefore greater efforts have been made to enlist the support of parents and to consult with them in the placement process. In practice this means that I will not confirm placements who are in voluntary care until the parents have given their permission and some commitment to the placement.

With younger teenagers it has been arranged for the parent or parents to meet the foster parents before the teenager so they can take responsibility for telling their son or daughter about the proposed placement. If parents and teenagers do not feel they have a say or any choice in the placement, why should they give it their full support when problems arise, as they inevitably will. Greater care is now given to the parents' part of the contract.

THEORETICAL BASIS FOR SPECIAL FOSTER CARE FOR ADOLESCENTS

Theories of social deviance and labelling were discussed above in the context of residential care tending to compound and not resolve problems. This final section develops three theoretical concepts which argue that family placement is logically and positively the best option for teenagers.

The first useful concept is that of identity formation developed by the psychiatrist Erikson (1968). Erikson saw life as a series of developmental stages, each one of which has to be negotiated successfully in order to have the capacity to move onto the next stage. The task for adolescence is to establish a coherent sense of identity in preparation for adult life. Failure to achieve this task leads to identity diffusion so that a person is faced by a number of possibly conflicting experiences which cannot be integrated.

As young people grow up they identify with their parents, then wider family, teachers, friends, and others. All contribute to an adolescent's sense of identity. Adolescence is a time when identity is particularly fluid and changeable. Some experimentation, even bizarre at times, allows the young person to try out different parts to add onto the basic core personality.

The difficulty for some young people in care comes when there is no basic core personality, or what there is has been deemed defective, inadequate or unacceptable. However, that "bad" aspect of personality has a history, has roots and does exist. To look at it is painful for a teenager, parent, and foster parent, but ignoring it does not make it go away. Although to ignore it may make life simpler for the social workers and other helpers, it does not help the teenager in care develop a coherent sense of who he or she is. The goal must be for all the teenager's past identifications to coexist in an entire, whole and consistent personality. There is evidence from studies on children of divorce that adolescents especially resent attempts to coerce them to take sides after their parents divorce, as they perhaps consciously try to integrate both sides of the family into an integrated personality (Mitchell, 1985; Piaget, 1981). There is a danger that the personality of a fostered teenager can develop in two or three isolated directions. Firstly, there is the identity which conforms to the expectations of the foster parents. While this identity can be quite persuasive and impressive, its roots and depth are suspect. Secondly, there is the identity which developed while at home which is very well rooted but may not be socially acceptable. Thirdly, many teenagers have what could be termed a "street identity," which is quite normal, usually not long-lived nor well-rooted, and will wither away of its own accord unless other points of identification are not available.

An actual case history of a teenager called Paul can illustrate the danger of developing a split identity. With the benefit of hindsight this case seems such an extreme example as to verge on a parody. However it's true. Paul came from a determinedly criminal family. His dad was a shady dealer, and his brothers stole. Paul was only fourteen and had a record as long as the proverbial arm. The magistrates were determined to teach him a lesson and lock him up, but they were persuaded to allow KFPS to work with him and provide him with different role models and a different peer group. He was placed in a foster family where the father is a policeman at the other end of the county. Paul settled well with his foster family, committed no crimes, went to school every day but went home less often. His parents never came to the foster home. There were occasional problems getting him back to the foster home on time after the visits home, but once he got there he was fine – it was too good to be true.

Paul sustained two different, and almost mutually exclusive identities for 18 months. In placement he was a model of upright and conforming youth, at home he reverted to being the Artful Dodger. He then committed such a succession of offences that even the impressive courtroom performance by his policeman/foster father did not prevent the inevitable. Paul's letters from Borstal to his foster parents expressed simply and movingly his crisis over identity. He did not know where he belonged; he had an acute case of identity diffusion.

How can KFPS help this process of identity formation? Firstly our model requires opportunities for important figures in the teenager's past and present to be incorporated into the fostering effort. If there is no continuity with the past, there can be no continuity of identity. If there is no continuity of identity, it is that much harder to give the young person on the threshold of leaving care the psychological robustness to survive.

Secondly our model usually provides two adult figures with whom the young person can identify. These figures are ever-present, consistent, caring and provide individual attention appropriate to the young person's needs. They do not change shifts, they are not subject to a forty-hour working week, and they do not change places of work as frequently as most social workers. They are consistent figures, and this encourages the adolescent's need for identification with adults. Given that identification with good role models is essential to the growth of a healthy identity, then it is difficult to conceive of means more suited than family placement to provide such models for adolescents, *especially* when these models actively seek to encourage the incorporation of previous role models (parents) into the adolescent's thinking.

The second major theorist whose writing is relevant is Piaget, who studied the intellectual development of children and adolescents. Most teenagers achieve a stage of thinking which is beyond the concrete and can take in abstract thought. Teenagers are learning to take a wider perspective, and part of this involves the ability to look at themselves in the light of their history. They learn to deal with abstract concepts like justice, morality, fairness, and to think their way through problems beforehand rather than stumble through in a state of bewilderment and surprise. This is not to say that teenagers always use this ability; in fact daily life in KFPS is replete with examples of abstract reasoning not being used. But its potential is there.

An illustration of the development of this type of thinking is Julie, whose mother was a prostitute. As a 14-year old her thinking was like a very young child. She did not want to think her mother was a prostitute, so she denied it. Her reality was "My mum is not on the game." Gradually the reality crept into her mind, despite vigorous efforts to shut it out. She then thought, "I am my mother's daughter, this is part of me," and she was indiscriminately promiscuous. Her thinking then developed so she could reason not only on the basis of concrete certainties, e.g., my mother is a prostitute, I am my mother's daughter, but also on the basis of hypotheses and suppositions. By being able to look at herself from the outside, she could consider abstractly, "What sort of woman do I want to be?" "Do I want to be like my mother?"

Once this intellectual stage is reached, time spent counseling and talking through alternatives is time well spent. Because the ability is often precarious, since it comes and goes as quickly as adolescent mood swings, it must be carefully nurtured by consistent discussion with the same caring adult. The ability to think through problems does not exist independently of a sympathetic environment in which this skill can be practiced.

The ability to think abstractly and to view oneself from the outside are prerequisites for being able to take responsibility for one's own decisions. Creating opportunities for teenagers to make their own decisions is most easily achieved given individual care. For example, to give permission for a seventeen-year old to stay out the night is possible if he or she is the only person in the immediate age group requesting the privilege. If he or she were in residential care, and there would be implications and possible unrest amongst a small group of sixteen-year olds, then the seventeen-year old is more likely to have to stay at home in the interests of the larger group. Allowing teenagers to make more of their own decisions and be accountable for the consequences is an essential step in their development, which requires individual care in the community, so that they are able to take the same risks as teenagers their age normally would.

A third theorist important to the KFPS is the English psychiatrist

Peter Bruggen. Bruggen argues (1975) that disturbed adolescents feel that they can run both their own family and society, and they demand to do so. They run beyond control and indulge in all sorts of behavior which is destructive to themselves and to society. He believes that many such adolescents are looking for limits, some structure to contain them, and someone to confront them within a relationship which shows concern for the individual adolescent. He argues for necessary confrontation and acceptance of the teenager's hostility because "It is easier to give in but disastrous in the long run."

The absence or confused lines of authority for teenagers in their own families is often a primary reason for them coming into care. The result of coming into care is often more confused lines of authority. Social service departments seem to exercise authority by committee, and the person in the committee with the least knowledge of the teenager often has the most power. The division of care (the daily looking after of the teenager) and control (the authority to make important decisions about the teenager) is peculiar to children in care, is stigmatizing to them, and, especially when applied to the particular phase of adolescence, can be very destructive. The KFPS model, for the most part, unites care and control. When an angry teenager is rowing with a foster parent and making demands on a Saturday night, it cannot wait for a committee decision the following week. By increasing the status of foster parents and providing them with specialized support staff, the authority to back the Saturday night decision is usually forthcoming. This unity of care and control is essential. It is not a characteristic unique to foster care; it can also be found in well-run residential homes where the personal status of the head of home means that his or her authority will prevail. However it is just common sense that the chances of achieving clear rules and authority are much greater between husband and wife than amongst a large group of care staff. The alternative to providing clear authority is to present teenagers with endless opportunities to play both ends against the middle, to try and divide and rule. This can postpone the day indefinitely when they must take responsibility for their own behavior.

In summary, the KFPS experience suggests that an understanding of the role of authority in adolescent disturbance, the growth of intellectual development and the development of identity at adolescence provide the relevant thinking to guide action which will be in the interests of the young people who come to us for both a practical and thoughtful service.

Chapter 5

Family Preservation in Foster Care: Fit or Fiction?

Peter W. Forsythe

ABSTRACT. Treatment foster care is described in respect to the permanency continuum, particularly the importance of family connectedness for children placed out of home. The placement of specialist foster care in the treatment continuum is identified along with the associated advantages and challenges to be met.

The central theme of this paper is that foster family care and treatment foster care are part of the permanency continuum and are not separate from that continuum. Permanency planning involves values and issues of definition. How these are understood will influence whether people think that treatment foster care fits on the permanence continuum. A few points will be made about what gets in the way of appropriate responses and decisions about removing children from parents when we are faced with treatment alternatives for families in trouble. I will stress the importance of expanding the response and having specialized foster care as one part of that expansion. Finally I will raise a series of issues and challenges that need to be addressed if special foster care is to be a responsible part of the permanency continuum.

Permanency planning developed to get more of the children caught in the public social service system adopted or returned to

Peter W. Forsythe is Vice President of the Clark Foundation, 250 Park Avenue, New York, NY 10017.

their pre-care families. Initial definitions were unduly restrictive. Only children under twelve were included in the original permanency planning project in Oregon. Time has taught us that this restriction was inappropriate, although there are still some lingering notions that permanency planning is not appropriate for adolescents. I believe that all people need family connections, including adolescents. "Family connectedness" may be a better term to use. We need to think of family connectedness as the core of permanency planning.

Family connectedness is an awkward phrase but I have not found a better one. It is not an absolute concept, but, like happiness, we want and ought to have as much of it as we can achieve. At the very least, just as we defend our right to the "pursuit of happiness" we should support a pursuit of permanency or family connectedness for all children, particularly those in substitute care. The degree of family connectedness of a child may be measured by cultural standards and by legal standards. Permanency planning or family connectedness is best measured by notions of what people have with their family ties. Legal recognition and protection, clear identity, good and dependable nurture, and so forth are what we all expect in the normal scheme of things. These are the same things we seek through family connectedness and permanency planning for those whose functional family ties have been disrupted by placement or by other circumstances or events. There is something fundamental about intergenerational connectedness for all of us; it is a lifelong need. Everybody needs family in one way or another at all times and phases of life.

Families are not just needed by children. The idea of a family connectedness hierarchy ought to be a part of our thinking. The bio-family is the source of permanence for most of us. Even when periodically we are frustrated and dislike our families, we usually carry on and provide for our children and maintain connectedness to that line from which we came. And when that doesn't work, the legal creation of family by adoption is next best. Adoption has the most characteristics of the biological family of any alternative recognized by society. Adoption is preferable to foster care because of what it means to be legally recognized as a family. Adoption comes closest to biological connectedness. It formalizes the commitments and expectations as well as the rights and the responsibilities that we all take for granted in normal family relations.

Everybody needs some kind of a connection, foster-parent, worker-cottage parent, teacher, friend, somebody to whom we can look. For children who have grown up in care we owe an obligation to help them connect to somebody. Don't overlook the bio-parents who may have been unable or unwilling to nurture and care for a child but may be able to have an important relationship reestablished, adult to adult, even after years of separation. The litmus test is who you call when you want to tell someone you're going to get married or you've just had a child. Where do you go when you want that kind of unqualified, intergenerational acceptance? In most instances, that's family. Family is the place where when you go they have to take you in. And we owe every child just such a place.

Sometimes permanence and connectedness is achieved by planning and sometimes by default. Sometimes it happens in spite of us. Even when it happens because of our benign neglect, it doesn't mean that benign neglect is excusable. Sometimes permanence is assisted and sometimes frustrated by the way we interact with families. In many instances we unwittingly do damage to the prospects of permanency for many children. Failing to make timely decisions, frustrating visitations, failing to facilitate or even permit parental participation in treatment, education or care decisions are all examples of ways we do damage to family connectedness.

Permanency planning is the skeleton of case planning and the backbone of good treatment. There are other issues that must be added to flesh out the whole plan, but a weak framework or skeleton fails to support our fundamental obligation of enhancing family connection.

Permanency planning, like practicing law, has a defect as a phrase. My kids used to say, "Well, you're practicing law, when are you really going to do it?" That is true with permanency planning; regardless of the words the essence is making it happen. The real goal of permanency is *doing* it, not simply planning for it. It calls for action and not just intention.

Permanency planning is central to the whole continuum of response to children in need of services. On the one hand it means the prevention of unnecessary dismemberment of a family, such as doing all one reasonably can to keep a family together while meeting the needs for treatment or service for its children. It means removing perpetrators and not victims. It means mounting intensive family preservation efforts before you can conclude that there are no alternatives to child removal. Reunification is always more difficult and problematic than family preservation. Like with Humpty Dumpty we are far better off not having to put the family back together. When placement is necessary, a central permanency principle is promoting parental involvement with children. Visitation, contact, involvement in treatment, participation in decisions – all of these things facilitate reunification. Whether it is specialized treatment or regular; whether it is short- or long-term, too often we fail to recognize the importance of family involvement. It's tough. It's inconvenient for staff. It's messy, uneven, and conflict-producing. Yet it is the key to the timely discharge to family with success or to the hard decisions toward termination of parental rights and then adoption.

Kids and adults have an enormous drive to get back to roots, to connect even with very dysfunctional families. A learned judge in Michigan is experimenting with restoring parental rights when no other family ties have been established for a child before discharge from care. His belief is that once the youth reached adulthood there is no reason why that person should be deprived of biological ties. The social concerns about parenting capacity are moot. When appropriate, this practice assists all involved to regain family connectedness.

The choices we make about timeliness, location and method of treatment for troubled children do affect permanency planning. How we respond, when we respond, and why we respond are all important to family connectedness. Removal from the family is a very important threshold. Removing a child from a family is like starting a large boulder rolling ever so slowly down an incline. You must not only slow down and stop the boulder but push it back uphill as you reconstruct and reconnect what you have put asunder. Often foster care or treatment foster care is appropriate, but even then something happens at the threshold of removal which has to then be rebuilt. If you compare success in preventing removal versus reconnecting or reunification, reunification is more difficult, problematic, and less likely to be sustained. There is a definite role for treatment foster care, but removal is an important threshold and the treatment choice made does affect the tasks we have to undertake in the success rate in permanency planning.

There is a football saying about throwing a forward pass; three things can happen and two of them are bad. When we remove a child, three or four or more things can happen, and several of them are bad. If we believe in family connectedness, we will be very careful about how we maintain ties and what we do with family connectedness during the period of removal. This awareness, concern, and response to family is central to fulfilling the promise of treatment foster care. Physical distance is an aggravating factor. Placement should be as close to family, neighborhood, friends, school, culture and community as possible. Only for exceptional reasons should we accept avoidable distance and then substantial compensation in program design is imperative. Concerns about restrictiveness and the impact of placement setting does motivate people to think of family-like settings. Such settings are close to home in terms of familiarity, if not geography. Geography is important, but specialized foster care offers less distance from the child's experiences than does a congregate living situation.

Coercion is another worrisome threshold. Coercion refers to the degree to which somebody imposes, interferes with, undermines, or takes away power, authority, and responsibility from the family to plan, make choices about, and deal with its children. Who proposed the placement? How is the service plan constructed? Have all reasonable services alternatives been considered, explored, and offered? These are all critical questions. And what of coercion? Much that is ostensibly voluntary is really coercive because parents receive a message that their views really don't count. No alternatives are offered. Whether in the form of a suggestion, implied threat, or court order, the degree and nature of coercion should be minimized and also recognized as an important aspect of treatment choices. It will usually affect the level of permanency that will be achieved in the future. Justifiable, or at least understandable, resistance to coercion will often show up in case records as "uncooperative family," or "refusal to acknowledge problems," or through misinterpretation or misrepresentation of parental behavior. Perhaps the resistance is tenacity, defense of family connectedness, and belief in the importance of keeping this child within the family structure. These strengths can be used and developed to support and rekindle family ties. These are strengths to be acknowledged, appreciated, and built upon as compared to the family that acquiesces and allows the child to be quietly taken away.

The values that undergird our work also effect treatment choices and permanency planning. Values may be expressed openly in our choices or can remain unexpressed but still reflected in the decisions we make—in our treatment approaches and in our caretaking arrangements. I believe that the underlying beliefs and values should be explicit, understood, intentional, and consistent throughout the program and also consistent with the ultimate goals. One value is family connectedness. If family connectedness is seen as the core of treatment planning, as the fundamental objective, it must be articulated, appreciated and supported by action. A related value is respect for the biological parents, adoptive parents or pre-care family. We owe respect for their potential and ultimate responsibility. We owe this in terms of a nonjudgmental approach that will maximize the opportunity for healing, learning, and growing. We owe a respect that understands that blame is complicated and in large part irrelevant. Adolescent struggles with parents over values often result in older children ending up in care. Is the youth at fault? Or is the parent neglectful? We need a no-fault procedure. Fault is not the issue. Determination of fault is difficult and usually counterproductive. Changing behaviors, teaching new skills, weathering the emotional crises—these are productive pursuits.

Belief in the capacity and desire of people to change is another important value. Families, however dysfunctional, do not generally enjoy their dysfunction. They would rather be well and better. Families who appear to be enjoying their dysfunctional situation probably see no viable alternative. Helping families to experience success with alternatives will cause them to wish to change, want to be different, and work to adapt to the pressures and at least the minimum standards of the law and society.

Another important value is promoting empowerment and avoiding dependency. At best, services are temporary interjections in the life of a person or family. Empowerment requires focusing on helping people solve problems for themselves. This requires openness, trust, and respect for family goals that are too often lost in the frustration of trying to deal with the dysfunction of a particular child and family. Is it our job to fix the family, or is it our job to enable the family to fix themselves? Your answer to this question will make a big difference in what service response is offered and how services are planned and delivered to or with the family members.

We ought to see presenting problems—the explosions and surface eruptions of family behaviors—as social aggravation indicators or behavior which makes society irritated at the moment. Running away from school, lying, cheating, truancy, and delinquent behavior are symptoms of more fundamental and common problems. Beneath the surface lies the material with which one can best work. Too often, we classify and categorize children and families on the basis of a presenting problem, only to find another problem, and then we call them "multi-problem" families. These are simply social irritation labels that can get in the way of more coordinated and comprehensive professional response. They divide us by diagnosis.

But what else inhibits our treatment choices on the permanency planning continuum? Personal considerations may lead us to make decisions that pass responsibility for the child or family to somebody else's caseload. Or we fail to make difficult decisions, such as to reunify a child and family, because we want to protect ourselves from the criticism of having made a mistake. We may avoid moving to terminate parental rights or to place a foster child for adoption because we shy away from the confrontation with bio-parents, foster parents, lawyers and judges that will be involved. We may experience resource limitations and blame the legislature or taxpayers, but in many instances we need to look to see whether even with resource issues there are things that we might do, like broaden our knowledge of alternatives. Some of this is really inertia, a predisposition to keep on doing what we have always done rather then consider alternative uses of current resources. A lack of flexibility often comes out of our limited sense of accountability and wanting things in pigeonholes with clear definitions and not trusting anybody to do anything which might be flexible or sensible but different. Are we prepared to trust and empower staff or each other just as we need to concentrate on empowering children and their families?

Another matter inhibiting appropriate treatment choices is diagnostic fads. We get caught labeling kids in a certain way or responding almost out of habit. We need more dialogue between child welfare, mental health, and juvenile justice to recognize "You call it that, we call it this, we diagnose them this way, you diagnose them that way, but they're mostly the same kids in families." There is an enormous overlap. Ignoring that fact, often we label families and children, and then we respond only in terms of often arbitrary and almost always oversimplified and child-focused labels. As a result, we unnecessarily inhibit and restrict the treatment choices we see, and the choices we make. Often labeling and restricting choice is the result of professional politics, vested interest, turf, and tradition. Acknowledging this can lead us on the path to action and correction.

Research on public attitudes about child abuse and neglect shows that most people believe removal from families is the best and only way to provide safety for children in such families. Professionals use the same equation. We try to protect a kid by taking him or her out of a family and putting them someplace else with little regard for family connectedness or alternative ways to protect them.

Community pressure is one of the reasons we are inhibited from making more appropriate treatment choices in these circumstances. Part of the reason for this is the undervaluing of family. We value your family or my family but "those" families we undervalue. People applaud family preservation goals, but then say, "You don't really mean keeping a kid in that kind of family, do you?" YES, that is what I mean. Family preservations is not a political slogan and it has not been captured by the right or the left, but is a thorough, complicated, internally held, and deeply rooted valuing of family.

Sometimes in our rescue fantasies we simply think our professional expertise and clinical judgement is better than family. Agencies have been known to think of themselves as families and to see themselves as a permanent family. Since almost all children ultimately leave placement and return to the real world without family, we must get beyond this short-sighted and counterproductive rescue mentality. Being family-like is not being family. It's good, but it's different.

We can do a lot of good in treatment, but we also ought to understand the limitations and our often unrealistic expectations of our ability to fix things. Many of us see our work as vaccination social work or vaccination treatment. Just take a dose of what we offer and you will be immune to problems in the future. Nonsense. Then there's another view that might be called intravenous treatment; if you just hook me up to my worker or therapist, and we drip in a little bit of good on an ongoing basis, you'll be just fine. But there is another alternative. We can see treatment as an episodic intervention. We can learn to set sensible and measurable goals, do what we can at this stage of family and child crisis or development, do as little harm as possible in the process, and once the equilibrium is reestablished or the crisis resolved, let the family function. They won't be a perfect television family but will have all the warts that real families have. When and if they need treatment or service in the future we should be ready and able to respond without a sense of failure that they weren't cured forever in the first place.

Professionals aren't the only answer to problems; we can and must do more to appreciate and facilitate the natural helping systems to which every successful family has access. Emergency responses also inhibit our choices. Many emergencies are simply the current name for yesterday's work undone. We didn't do what we should have and the result is an emergency.

The treatment continuum does need expansion and specialized foster care is an important new element. Interest should also be focused on expanding the front end of the continuum with family preservation services and new kinds of prevention that is articulate about what we are preventing and how. When one looks at the placement portion of the services continuum, specialized foster care is toward the front end. We need to identify ways in which family foster care can be more family centered and have the intensity and treatment tools to provide effective care for children and youth in family settings without moving them to more restrictive settings. Specialized treatment families or treatment foster care is to family foster care what residential treatment centers are to the orphanage. If treatment foster care can retain a family atmosphere, provide a community base, and provide for bio-family connectedness and involvement, it can be an even more effective learning laboratory for children and youths.

Treatment foster care can expand and contract with ease and

speed. It does not have the rigidity of bricks and mortar that cripples the ability to adapt to changes in demand. But there are some limitations, and they need to be carefully considered. Treatment foster care may be cheaper and better than residential treatment centers, but one needs to be very conscious of the net widening risks. We must not use treatment family care for children who ought not be in any kind of out-of-home care.

There are also some issues and challenges for treatment foster care to explore in greater depth as it develops. They are a challenge to the movement and its leaders to give greater substantive measuring to the term "treatment foster care." It can't just be anything anybody does other than regular foster care. And yet at the same time, a rigid definition that excludes further development and creativity or mandates cookie cutter replication won't benefit development either.

A second challenge is to articulate the technology, values, treatment theories, and approaches so that evaluation can tease out what makes a difference. In so-called home-based care, the idea has developed that it doesn't make any difference how the service is delivered. All approaches are equally good. Poppycock! Choices do make a difference. They may be better for one family or another kind of family, they may be cheaper, they may be less intrusive, they may be more suited to a particular professional training or working climate, but they do make a difference. We need to focus on different approaches and explore them, figure out what's good, what's bad, what's useful, when it's good, and when it's bad. Treatment foster care needs to be a concept, an idea that has substance and can be described, evaluated and replicated.

Family connectedness is also a challenge. There is too little in the current treatment foster care literature about staying connected with the biological family. Providing a liaison worker is not enough. What are family responsibilities, what are family rights, and what is the integral connection? In New York, Dr. Salvador Minuchin is training foster parents in three agencies to be much more sensitive about and responsive to bio-families. One way is to stop having workers as intermediaries between foster and biological parents and to increase the direct contact between them. The two families will be working together. The foster family will be the connection, a model, and a support to bio-families.

There are collateral issues like length of stay, and therefore, costs. Per diem is not a useful measures of cost. Full case costs are what to worry about. The per diem times length of stay equals cost. Comparisons of alternatives need to be made in that way with adjustments for outcome. What is success? There needs to be some sharpening in our thinking about what we consider successful. Moving to a less restrictive placement is not a sufficient definition. A last challenge is to increase the retention of gains made in the treatment family after return home. Not enough attention is given to that. It may be the bottom line.

Treatment foster care has a marvelous potential to expand the continuum of care and to meet the needs of some children and their families in new settings with flexibility that hasn't existed in the past. It will only reach its full potential as treatment foster care becomes part of the permanency continuum and addresses the fundamental need of every child for a family connection.

Chapter 6

Northern Ireland as a Case Study of the Development of Treatment Foster Care

Mary McColgan

ABSTRACT. Major developments in the history of fostering in Northern Ireland are described, major problems identified and suggestions made for the current and future development of specialist fostering arrangements.

Foster care in Northern Ireland is regarded as an integral part of child care services. It has a legislative basis which has roots in the Poor Law and the emphasis in fostering has been on the provision of "substitute parenting" for children in care. Statutory and voluntary agencies have increasingly come to recognize the limitations of the traditional concept of foster care as a means of dealing with the complex needs of children who are received into the care system. This paper traces some of the important historical factors which influenced the development of this traditional approach and examines the role of traditional fostering and its influences on child care policy and practice. Finally the paper explores the emergence of professional fostering as an approach to foster care which attempts to help children resolve their difficulties in addition to providing primary care within a family setting.

Mary McColgan is Lecturer in Social Work, Department of Applied Social Studies, University of Ulster, Magee College, Northland Road, Derry BT52, Northern Ireland.

A point to be borne in mind is that the whole of Ireland was subject to social legislation passed by British Parliament (Westminster) from the Act of Union in 1800 until 1921. The Government of Ireland Act in 1920 established a separate Northern Ireland Government and parliament which came into effect in 1921. This meant that Northern Ireland had its own parliament and was responsible to a large degree for the development of its own social legislation. The British Government retained reserve powers for a range of responsibilities which did not include legislation in the field of social welfare. Thus Northern Ireland experienced a high and increasing degree of legislative as well as administrative autonomy in relation to social legislation and this situation continued until direct rule in 1972. Since then all Norther Ireland legislation is dealt with at Westminster by virtue of "Orders in Council." In effect this has meant that legislation is subject to limited debate and cannot be amended once it has been presented to the House of Commons (Birrell and Murie, 1981).

Another important point is that, although Northern Ireland's social legislation appeared to practice parity in relation to British legislation, there were wide divergences in practice, particularly in relation to education, housing, and child welfare. For example, child care legislation in Northern Ireland has retained a strong focus on the family. The Southern Government by comparison has had total independence for its social legislation since 1921 but continued to operate under the pre-1921 British legislation until a relatively recent major review of its personal services social legislation.

Fostering is part of a range of child care services which are provided by personal social services against a background of a number of enactments. This legislation provides care for children and young people from birth to the age of 18 years and also care for their families. While a significant role is played in these services by the voluntary sector, the Health and Social Services Boards in Northern Ireland have a statutory obligation to safeguard the interests of children and assist families and children in certain ways. This response to child care is the result of a reorganized structure of health and personal social services which was operationalized on October 1, 1973. The reorganization in Northern Ireland brought together the three separate branches of the health services — hospital, general

practitioners, and local health authority—within a unified administration. The three branches of the personal social services—local
welfare services, social work within the health service, and social
work for the mentally subnormal—were also brought together in
partnership with the health service and within the same administrative framework (Craigavon, The Decision Partnership, 1978). The
inclusion of the personal social services in the same administrative
structure is the most significant difference between reorganization
in the Province and that of England, Wales, and Scotland.

The key authorities within the new organization are the Department of Health and Social Services, the Area Boards, and the District Units of Management. The Department of Health and Social
Services is responsible for overall objectives, policies and resource
allocation, the Area Boards for planning and monitoring of services
and the District Units for managing and delivering services.

The Concise Oxford Dictionary defines foster care thus: "To
tend affectionately, cherish, promote the growth of." Such positive
aspects have not always underlined the fostering concept. A historical perspective highlights the emergence of foster care through various phases with emphasis on work, religion, and education. During
Tudor times, for example, fostering was regarded as a method of
meeting the needs of pauper children, but the work ethic dominated
this period.

By the early and mid-nineteenth century, children were being
exploited as workers during the Industrial Revolution. Concerns for
the plight of such children were led by Barnardo and Shaftsbury,
who worked as "child savers" among destitute children placed in
Parish workhouses. In England particularly the twin themes of education and religion began to replace the work principle as a guide to
the needs of the young (Central Personal Social Services Advisory
Committee, 1980).

By contrast, there is an interesting historical precedent for fostering in Ireland. Both prior and during the Norman era, fosterage, as
it was identified, played an important part in Irish social organization. Fathers often sent their sons to be reared with other families
or, after the arrival of Christianity, with a priest or religious community. Bonds created often influenced allegiance in later life even
at political levels. Under the old Irish code of law, there were two

kinds of fostering, one for affection, the other for payment. The relationship created could only be dissolved by death, crime, marriage, or entry into the religious community (Marron et al., 1982).

The Poor Law of 1838 had seen the creation of workhouses to care for the needs of the destitute and poor. These workhouses were administered by a Board of Guardians and even at that stage, the poor or destitute had no statutory right to relief. The roots of present day legislation in relation to fostering lie in the Poor Law Amendment Act of 1862. In an attempt to recognize that the workhouse atmosphere was not suitable for children and to deal with the high mortality rates of infants who were admitted to the workhouse without their mothers, the Act empowered the Board of Guardians "to place any orphans or deserted child out of the workhouse if they shall think fit to do so, by placing such child out at nurse" (Central Personal Social Services, 1980). An age limit of five years was set, but this could be extended to include children up to eight years.

Subsequent legislation sought to improve the situation of children in deprived circumstances. Noteworthy among this was the Orphans and Deserted Children (Ireland) Act 1876 which extended the age up to which children could be fostered to 13 years. This act also represented the first step in what later became Boarding-Out Regulations with its emphasis on the duties of foster-parents: cleanliness (the child was to be washed at least once every day), shelter, food and clothing, medical attention, schooling, church attendance. A receiving officer appointed to supervise these situations was obliged to visit the child once a month and to keep a written record of each visit (Herron and Caul, 1980). The Pauper Children Acts of 1898 and 1902 defined the classes of children eligible for boarding-out and permitted the then local government boards to fix the age limit. The effect of this legislation led to a decrease in the proportion of children under 15 years of age in the workhouse. For example, the proportion of children to total residents in 1872 was 25.5% and by 1902 this had dropped to 13.1% (Herron and Caul, 1980). This preference for fostering as an alternative to residential care is a theme which continues even to the present day and will be explored further.

By the turn of the century, the Poor Law legislation was in disarray and the situation was reviewed by two Poor Law Commissions of 1906 and 1909. Having surveyed the population of the work-houses, the Commission of 1906 made recommendations for ten categories of people, including infants and children. Their report contained far sighted provisions for fostering, but their reasons were often practical rather than emotional. They recognized that "Boarding out . . . is also the cheapest mode of rearing children" (Herron and Caul, 1980). They advocated boarding-out as a way of dealing with effects of institutionalized behavior. "Not being used to small houses and to common place life . . . institution-reared children were found to be awkward and out of their element when placed among ordinary surroundings." Having been reared in institutions, "children . . . were thought to be not tough or hardy as children brought up in ordinary houses. . . ." The subsequent Commission of 1909 was cautious about wholesale fostering and wished its merits to be "more fully investigated and to be assured of the supply of adequate foster parents" (Herron and Caul).

The 1908 Children Act had far-reaching effects in Ireland. It consolidated and amended earlier legislation relating to child life protection; defined neglect as failure to provide food, clothing, medical aid or lodgings, made it an offense to willfully assault, neglect, ill-treat or abandon a child or young person in a manner likely to cause suffering or injury to health and gave courts the power to commit the children to the care of a relative or other "fit person" (Evason, 1976). This act remained the principal legislation from the formation of the state of Northern Ireland in 1921 until 1950. It is still the principal act in relation to children and young persons in the Republic of Ireland. The significant feature of this act was its concentration on the offense of the parent rather than the needs of the child. This preoccupation with inadequate or "unfit" parenting is still a pervasive theme in current legislation. This development has been significant in determining the role of fostering as fulfilling a "substitute parenting" role in relation to children who are unable to be cared for by parents.

The 1950 Children and Young Persons Act (Northern Ireland) stipulated that residential care was only to be provided for children where "it is not practicable or desirable for the time being to make arrangements for boarding-out" (Central Personal Social Services, 1980). This commitment in favor of fostering as the best form of substitute care reflected the thinking of the 1946 Curtis Committee in England and the Northern Ireland legislation was accompanied by statutory rules and orders defining procedures required in approving and maintaining contact with foster homes. In addition, welfare authorities were requested to report to the Ministry of Home Affairs if children had not been boarded-out within three months. Under the 1950 act, a child welfare council was established to advise the ministry of matters affecting the welfare of children and young persons.

A report compiled by the Child Welfare Council in 1956 echoed the importance of family life for children in residential care. They felt that the child in care ". . . has a right to a house of his own and the happiness and security of normal family life." They suggested that adoption was the best method of providing this house with security, but if that was not possible, then ". . . boarding-out is considered the best alternative." If legislation advocated boarding-out, then social work practice was beginning to reflect this in its commitment to boarding-out. By 1959-60 the total number of children in the care of local authorities was 1148. Of these 724 were boarded-out, 226 were in welfare authority residential homes, and 152 were maintained in voluntary homes on behalf of welfare authorities.

Statistics for the same period from the voluntary sector reflect a decline in the number of children in voluntary homes (751). However, apart from children in Dr. Barnardo's care, voluntary homes rarely arranged boarding-out. In fact, Dr. Barnardo had instigated enlightened fostering practices as early as 1866 when the Auxiliary Board-out scheme had been created for assisting mothers with illegitimate babies. This scheme enabled children to be fostered within easy travelling distance so that the mother could maintain contact and keep direct responsibility for the child's upbringing. There were rigidly enforced requirements with regard to regular existing and consistent payment of expenses. The penalty for failure to uphold these requirements was the immediate threat to withdraw the child from the foster home.

Some of the final recommendations of the Child Welfare Council Report highlight the strong religious stencil which has tended to be stamped over discussions on social issues in Northern Ireland. It reinforced the importance of allocating children to foster homes in line with their religious backgrounds. Although this question of religious upbringing was also embodied in English legislation, this preoccupation is still a feature of current legislation and practice.

The legislation enacted in the 1968 Children and Young Persons Act (Northern Ireland) introduced a preventive child care element. Local authorities were given discretionary power to assist families materially or with cash payment to prevent children being received into care. The act identified a number of situations where children and young persons are regarded as potentially vulnerable, and it outlined what could constitute acceptable practice and procedures. With relation to boarding-out, the legislation confirmed the need to "approve" households where children were to be placed. This approval was governed by regulations which stipulated that children had to be boarded-out with a person ". . . of the same religious persuasion as the child or gives an undertaking that the child will be brought up in that religious persuasion."

The desirability of boarding-out was stressed where practical and desirable and reinforced the primacy given to fostering by legislation. The Boarding-Out Regulations of 1976 elaborated on this, outlining procedures and practices in relation to children who were to be boarded-out with foster parents. Briefly the boards had an additional duty in relation to children boarded-out by voluntary organizations. They had to satisfy themselves that the organization was in a position to supervise the placement satisfactorily, or if not, the board was empowered to take over and perform such duties. In practice the four boards have established practices which have been negotiated with voluntary agencies, and these are rarely the subject of contention.

This emphasis on the primacy of fostering in legislation was reviewed by the Black Committee (Children and Young Persons Review Group, 1977) which had as its brief the review of children and young persons legislation and the future structure of the Probation Service in Northern Ireland. They acknowledged the importance of fostering as a feature of child care policy and emphasized that the fostering task was not simply a substitute for the parent/child relationship but a difficult and demanding task which may require foster parents to work with the child's natural family in a situation which could give rise to conflict. The committee was concerned about the "tug of war" situations some children and foster parents experienced and recommended the concept of custodianship as envisaged by the 1975 Children's Act of England. This would offer foster parents legal custody of their foster child without recourse to adoption. The committee's recommendations underline the permanency issues in fostering. This emphasis has also been challenged by the 1980 Sub-Committee on Foster Care in Northern Ireland. Their report has been highly critical of this practice on the basis that the emphasis on boarding-out is unjustified. Rather they hold the view that "it is a professional decision which form of care is most appropriate for an individual child."

No discussion of fostering in Northern Ireland would be complete without reference to the political and civil unrest and its implication for fostering. The period in question spans from 1969 to date and is referred to as the "troubles." It must be emphasized that the troubles, although referred to as if they were an entity, are in effect a complex series of events which range from riots where families were intimidated out of their homes, the introduction of internment, "no go" areas, hunger strikes, and bombings to present day assassinations of security and civilian personnel. All this has happened against a backdrop of high unemployment, high levels of poverty, and a level of socioeconomic deprivation which is higher than other parts of the United Kingdom.

Research into the effects of the troubles on the welfare of children and child welfare services are not widely documented (Kelly, 1979). Powell (1980) has noted that the children in Northern Ireland have to cope with violence arising out of the conflict in addition to the interconnected violence of severe deprivation. He cautioned that the emerging picture is more complex than the casual observer informed by media might expect. For example, although many children experienced acute anxiety reactions to the conflict, relatively few suffered from pathological symptoms. Truancy levels were not overall significantly higher than other parts of the United Kingdom. Further research studies reviewed in 1983 (Harbinson, p. 142) suggested that "relative normality seems to prevail in Northern Ireland — but within the now well established framework of political and sectarian violence." Equally it proposed that in the midst of severe social, economic, security and political problems ". . . children and young people are proving encouragingly adaptive" (Harbinson, p. 143).

The most important contribution of these studies has been to highlight two prevalent sets of beliefs about the "troubles." On the one hand is a set of beliefs usually held by outside observers, that the conflict and violence must have produced severely damaging long-term effects on people and children. The other view which seems to reflect insiders' observations is that the children who have grown up with the violence as a backdrop to their lives are resilient, adaptable, and have coped with the troubles. The authors emphasize that such assumptions cannot be proven or disproven but are open to further empirical tests.

In relation to the troubles and fostering, it is significant that to date no major research has been carried out in this area. Personal experience and discussions with social workers in Northern Ireland would lead me to speculate that the impact is not as great as one would imagine. However, there are a number of situations where the effects of the troubles can be considered to have implications for fostering and foster parents. For example, a proportion of approved foster parents may have links with the security forces, i.e., by virtue of employment as members of the Royal Ulster Constabulary, the Ulster Defence Regiment, or within the Prison Service. Clearly in the light of recent development such families experience tension and stress by virtue of the risks to which security forces are currently exposed. Any foster child placed within such a foster home would be unable to avoid the concomitant security vigilance which must be taken. This also has implications for parental contact with a child in such a foster home.

"Fostering is not in itself a single identifiable method of care. It offers a range of placements which have in common only the fact that they provide care in a family setting" (Working Party, 1976). The range of fostering includes the following:

1. Long-term — defined as a period exceeding six months;
2. Short-term — defined as lasting from one week to six months depending on family circumstances;

3. Emergency — defined as placement in crisis and at very short notice;

4. Pre-adoption fostering for new born babies prior to placement with adoptive parents;

5. Aunt and uncle schemes offering children in care some contact with family life on weekends or during day outings;

6. Five-day fostering — defined as alternative care during the week with return home at weekends; and

7. Care for adolescents — defined as short-term placements, for adolescents who are having problems at home.

The family setting is regarded as offering the child a chance to be part of a family unit and to have an alternative experience of family life with "loving parental figures." Foster parents are expected to do a difficult job of caring for a child as if it were a member of their family, and in acknowledgement of this role foster parents sign an undertaking which firmly places them in a substitute parent role. However the anomaly in this situation is that the Health and Social Services Boards entrust twenty-four hour care to foster parents and yet retain the authority and responsibility of all the decision making within the agency. Foster parents are unable to sign consents to medical treatment and can experience the removal of a child without prior discussion.

Much of the literature about fostering has stressed the foster parents' difficulties in understanding their role (Parker, 1966). Confusion has arisen when they are asked by agencies to think of themselves as substitute parents but then asked to assume the role of caretaker or therapist. Jane Rowe has captured the dilemma accurately when she reflects "In reality a foster parent's role . . . is always a combination of caretaker, therapist, compensatory parent and substitute parent" (Rowe, 1980). She suggests that the mix will vary according to the type of placement and may change throughout the duration of the child's stay in the foster home. She further contends that foster parents face a difficult task as they try "to fill in the gaps" of the parental role in a triangular relationship which involves natural parents, foster parents, and the agency all carrying some responsibility for the child. The foster parents' task is to ensure that the child's needs are met "without unnecessary overlapping of function" (Rowe, p. 58).

This task has been further complicated by a traditional assessment and selection procedure which Health and Social Services Boards have adopted as their practice. On the basis that fostering has been regarded primarily as providing "substitute parenting," the assessment model has been based on the premise that applicants either have or do not have the necessary characteristics and qualities to make successful foster parents. Further, there is an assumption that skilled social work investigation by a qualified social worker can select successful applicants who will pass the test. Extracts from the Western Health and Social Services Board's guidelines outline the following as essential fostering parenting skills:

1. The ability to provide love.
2. A high level of tolerance.
3. An understanding of the physical and emotional needs of children.
4. The ability to provide a child with a stable home environment.
5. The ability to provide sufficient stimulation to help a child's growth and development.

The focus in assessment is very much on the motives for fostering, marital relationship, childhood experiences, and parenting skills. Combined with medicals, personal references, and a check of criminal records, it is little wonder that most foster parents regard the experience as gruelling. R. Smith (1984) discusses this procedure and points out that if social workers see their task in terms of assessment and selection, "they will seek information from applicants as a basis for judging their suitability" (Smith, p. 79). She advocates a process of preparation and education which presupposes that the prospective applicants have the capacity to understand the tasks essential to fostering, can be helped to anticipate how they will deal with problems, can learn alternative methods of communication, and essentially have developed sufficient self-awareness to assess their own expectations and needs. The crucial difference in the two models is that in the latter the social worker helps the applicants make the choice for themselves. It also acknowledges that foster parents by virtue of their life experiences possess some of the qualities necessary for the fostering task and have the potential to develop. Because they have skills already, they have something to offer a partnership relationship.

A basic problem for most social workers is that they have not yet resolved the issue of whether foster parents are clients or partners in this caring relationship. Smith suggests this because of the foster parents' "peculiarly dual nature of initially requesting, but later providing, a specific kind of service." Developing foster parents' potential to provide this service is dependent partly on a social work attitude which acknowledges competence to undertake the task, practice which reflects this, and training which enables foster parents to develop their skill and expertise. Alongside this there has to be access to information, open communication, involvement in decision making, and working to agreed contracts.

It is really only in the last decade that recognition of this partnership role has emerged or that the training needs of foster parents have been identified. This has been evident in the increased use of Parenting Plus as a training method, the emergence of the Northern Ireland Foster Care Association which has encouraged the "colleague" relationship between social worker and foster parent, and the emergence of professional foster care projects. This development has coincided with a growing realization to deal with the needs of particular groups like adolescents and children who have been sexually abused.

Such a professional fostering scheme has been devised and developed by Dr. Barnardo's (Barnardo's, 1985), a voluntary agency whose aim is to recruit, train, and support foster families for children who would otherwise remain in children's homes or training schools. The project aims to finalize the "bringing up" of young adolescents who are referred to or labelled as "disturbed." Their definition of "bringing up" as combining the resolution of personal and behavioral problems with the giving of "normal" childhood and adolescence encapsulates the concept of treatment. Such an ethos is reflected in Masud Hoghughi's paper (1985) to the National Foster Care Association in 1984. He identifies a series of steps for dealing with a child who experienced problems. Hoghughi defines problems as "unacceptable conditions" which could be divided into physical, cognitive, family and home, social skills, antisocial behavior and personal problems. He suggests a logical sequence for dealing with these problems: referral, management, care, assessment, and treatment. Treatment was concerned with ameliorating the problem condition. He proposes that

> Fostering is used as a means of reducing the extent and intensity of that unacceptable condition and bringing it within our society's tolerance. This process of alleviating or remedying a condition so that it is no longer unacceptable is how we define "treatment" and is, therefore, the focal purpose of all fostering. (Hoghughi, p. 18)

This is clearly not a view which has been adopted wholeheartedly in relation to fostering in Northern Ireland. The professional fostering schemes appear to have developed to meet a "specialized" need, and the treatment element is not regarded as the basis of all forms of fostering.

It is significant that advances in professional fostering within Northern Ireland have been pioneered by the voluntary sector, particularly Dr. Barnardo's. The agency's scheme commenced in 1979 and was the first developed in Northern Ireland. It was based on the Kent Family Placement Project and was underpinned by a philosophy which regarded foster parents as part of a team which shaped the aims and tasks of providing "care and guidance" (defined as a fusion of social work intervention and appropriate caring). The project's intention was to provide an alternative family setting, primary care, a community, and an individualized plan which would "secure" the child and promote the potential for independence and fulfilled adulthood. Foster parents were recruited for "hard to place" older children, their work was regarded as task centered, and they were paid a fee for the job—£5600 per year in addition to normal boarding-out allowances and expenses for the maintenance of each child. The project has responsibility for the recruitment and training of foster parents and the supervision and support of the placement.

The initial intention to provide professional foster care for "hard to place" 12- to 18-year olds in residential homes or training schools led to referrals from Health and Social Services Boards and the Northern Ireland Office. The project has achieved its initial aim of placing twelve young people with professional foster parents. The strengths of the scheme have involved (1) a recognition of closely assessed matches between families and young people; (2) the training and support offered to foster parents; and (3) careful placement pre-planning which involves an individualized care plan for each child, established aims and objectives, and areas of particular focus for attention.

In recent years, in line with Dr. Barnardo's philosophy of implementation and evaluation, those involved in the project have proposed an extension of the professional foster home scheme. They see future expansion in terms of additional placements up to a maximum of 20 to meet the needs of young people in the 12 to 16 age group for whom foster care would be a viable alternative to residential or custodial care. They envisage a continuum of care which includes after-care services, and they are clear that the work involves evaluation "to provide information on the statutory authority and others considering the potential use and development of family placement" (Barnardo's, N.D.). They also regard professional fostering as a potential way of providing care for some mentally handicapped children.

Although Dr. Barnardo's has been at the forefront of professional fostering in the province, the area boards have also developed schemes of their own based on the Barnardo's project. The subjective opinion of some social workers is that this response appears to be motivated more by efforts to achieve cost effectiveness than to develop better fostering practice. Current costs to boards per child run to £172 per week. The various schemes which have been set up are currently located mainly in the Eastern Health and Social Services Board, notably South, North and West Belfast, North Down, and Ards. The scheme, for example, in North and West Belfast was developed four years ago in response to teenagers who had been in residential homes and who were regarded as "hard to place." Before these initiatives such children in similar situations had been referred to the Barnardo's project. As this scheme has also met its initial aims, its future expansion is aimed at providing professional foster care for younger children. Recent developments in the Southern Board have led to a proposal for a "Fee Paid Placement Scheme" (Southern Health and Social Services Board, 1987) to meet needs which are not being met by traditional and short-term placements. These needs exist because of several factors.

1. The age of the child (11 years to 17 years old).
2. Sibling groups of two or three for placement.
3. Children who have difficult and well-established behavior patterns, e.g., sexually overt behavior or extreme antisocial behavior as a result of severe physical or emotional deprivation or similar behavior as a result of fostering disruption.

Such "fee paid" foster parents could offer task-centered care to adolescents preparing to leave care, respite care where time out is needed from a placement or even from home, or care for a pregnant girl or adolescent mother with child. The potential range is wide, but the distinct difference is that the "fee paid placements" would be asked "to do a specific piece of work which traditional placements would not appear to wish to take on." These differences include the possibility of lack of reward for the task in return for offering some experience of normal family life.

While the emergence of these schemes is commended, it must be recognized they are not province-wide and those in operation seem to be developing in an uncoordinated idiosyncratic fashion. What does appear to be a common factor is that each scheme is attempting to model its practice on Dr. Barnardo's project, suggesting "variations on a theme." In reality the Barnardo's team has not been encouraged to provide training for these specialist schemes nor to pass on its expertise and knowledge in any formal way. It appears that social services staff who coordinate these schemes have merely spent some time informally discussing the mechanics of the project.

Reasons for this failure to achieve a coordinated response to professional fostering are varied. On the one hand, there is a body of opinion which believes that *all* foster parents are doing a professional job and that it is hypocritical to call some "professional" because they are receiving a fee. Others have reservations about the way such schemes are advertised, and this has led to fostering being considered a contentious term. What is perhaps closer to the truth are the ambivalent views held by social workers towards foster parents and vice versa, a lack of empirically-based local data, and finally social services boards who are both resistant to the concept of professional fostering and to utilizing the contribution of a voluntary organization which has been innovative in its development of professional fostering.

What is required is a forum for these organizations to share widely their evaluation of these experiments so that others may learn from them. In this way the needs of children in care can best be met by the development of an integrated system of services which recognizes that a pluralist approach involving both statutory and voluntary organizations is the best way of promoting effective care for children and their families.

For the present in Northern Ireland it seems that we are at a crossroads in terms of professional fostering. It is under-developed, under-utilized, and its potential under-recognized. The future lies in a coordinated, integrated, and planned response to its development.

PART II:
PROGRAM ISSUES

Chapter 7

The Sexually Abused Child
in Specialized Foster Care

Emily Jean McFadden

ABSTRACT. Placing sexually abused children in untrained foster homes creates risk that these children will again be victimized because their distorted patterns of communication and behavior will be misunderstood by the foster parents or typical patterns of touching within families will be misunderstood by the sexually abused child. Foster parents of sexually abused children require training to understand the message sexually abused children have typically received from their environments, the nature of sexual abuse as a progression of events as well as the context of the specific abuse experience of the child being placed, the difference between male and female abuse victims, typical behavioral patterns of sexually abused children and how to manage these behaviors in light of the developmental needs of all children, and to be able to structure family activities in a way that sets clear boundaries to both protect the foster child as

Emily Jean McFadden is Associate Professor at the Social Work Department of Eastern Michigan University, Ypsilanti, MI 48197.

well as the foster parents. Foster parents need to understand how to assist the child in learning how to appropriately express sexuality and to live comfortably within a family setting.

The child who has been sexually abused is at high risk in foster care placement. Such a child brings a repertoire of behaviors which appear to the untrained observer to be sexualized. These behaviors trigger a range of uneasy feelings in foster parents and challenge any unresolved issues they may have about their own sexuality. Because of such behaviors, children who have been sexually abused are at high risk for further maltreatment in their foster homes (McFadden, Stovall, 1984). The sexualized, seductive behaviors which they have learned as a means of pleasing adults may be misread by foster parents as an invitation. The same behaviors, particularly those involving aggression toward a smaller child, can provoke physical abuse as foster parents struggle to control unacceptable behavior. Other non-sexualized behaviors, such as wetting and soiling which are fairly typical of children who have been sexually abused, are behaviors which also lead to foster parent maltreatment (McFadden, Ryan, 1986). Many adults have residual negative feelings about sexuality, especially child sexuality. It is one thing for foster parents to understand intellectually that children who have been sexually abused may act out sexually (Brandt & Tisza, 1979) — it is entirely another matter when foster parents walk into a bedroom and see nine-year-old Sally performing fellatio on their infant son.

Inappropriate placements, failure to train foster parents, and failure to monitor the home are all correlated with foster care maltreatment (Miller, 1982). Such children are at high risk and desperately in need of the services which specialized foster care can provide. They are at great risk in untrained foster homes.

The life experiences of children who have been sexually abused require supportive treatment to undo the effects of life in a sexually abusive family and to ameliorate the profound underlying emotional neglect which almost always precedes the actual sexual abuse incidents. Treatment in this context refers to a working alliance between foster parents and therapist, focused on correcting the child's developmental deficits, teaching new and healthier lessons about family living, and helping the child to handle and resolve ambivalent and frightening feelings about the incidents and the perpetrator(s) (McFadden, 1986; Mrazek & Kempe, 1981). While treatment of the perpetrator and/or family system is paramount, such a discussion is beyond the scope of this article and has been widely explored elsewhere (Mrazek & Kempe, 1981; Justice and Justice, 1979; Dixon & Jenkin, 1981; and Mayer, 1983).

The purpose of this article is to delineate some of the issues which foster parents must understand in order to provide specialized foster care to children who have been sexually abused. These concepts can be shared with foster parents through training (McFadden, 1986; Dawson, 1985; Cunningham, 1982) and reinforced through support group discussion and one-on-one casework practice by the child's social worker or therapist. Foster parents must fully realize the risks to these children, and the risks they bring to the foster home before they can take the steps to provide a safe and therapeutic environment in which the child can heal and grow.

THE WORLD OF THE SEXUALLY ABUSED CHILD

All members of the treatment team, foster parents, workers, and therapists need to be aware of the implications of the messages children have received in the environments in which they are sexually victimized. Some messages are obvious:

— Children are supposed to please adults.
— Children please adults when they behave in a sexual way.
— Children aren't allowed to talk about the sexual things that happen.
— Children's feelings don't count.

Other messages are more subtle:

— Children are powerless.
— Children have a strange power that makes adults go out of control.
— You can't ask for what you need.
— You can't expect to get what you need unless you behave sexually.

— The world is a frightening place.
— People abandon other people unless their sexual needs are met.
— Adults have a right to do whatever they want to children.
— If adults don't get what they want they might abandon or hurt children.
— Parents don't protect children.
— Children have to do whatever adults want them to do.
— Children can't feel or express their feelings.

Almost all sexually abused children have common problems. They were emotionally neglected prior to the sexual abuse incidents. If they had been protected by at least one parent; if they had learned to respect their own bodies and to say "no"; if they have been provided with adequate supervision; if they had received normal love and nurturing; if they had been encouraged to communicate openly with their parent(s), then in all likelihood the sexual abuse would not have occurred or would have been stopped after the first incident when the child complained to the protecting parent.

Emotional neglect is compounded by survival threats and distortions of reality which often accompany sexual abuse (Damon, Todd & McFarlane, 1987). Many perpetrators exploit the child's fear of abandonment and claim that the child's cooperation is the only thing keeping the perpetrator from leaving the family. A few perpetrators use threats of bodily harm to ensure the child's complicity. Others draw on the child's protectiveness of siblings, arguing compellingly that the child's cooperation will protect siblings from sexual maltreatment. While threats render children anxious beyond any manageable extent, denial distorts the child's perception of reality. The child knows all too well the sexual abuse is real, yet denial by the perpetrator and accusations that the child is lying cause great confusion, and ultimately undermine the child's confidence in reality testing. It is easy for foster parents to understand that the sexual abuse when combined with emotional neglect can lead to serious emotional disturbance for the child.

What is not as clear and needs to be spotlighted for foster parents is the manner in which the child's previous experience affects his or her adjustment to the foster home and colors perceptions of the foster family. The intimacy and touching of normal family life are confusing and appear to involve sexual content to a child whose only physical nurturing came through sexual contact. Such a child is aware of the progression of activities which led up to an actual sexual contact and does not know how to differentiate that which is sexual from that which was part of the seduction:

> Tom, a nine-year-old in foster care, had been involved with a pedophile who had taken pornographic pictures. His friend had first engaged Tom by hiring him to sweep out the front of his shop. Tom was pleased to earn the extra money. The perpetrator then gained Tom's confidence by spending a lot of time talking to Tom about his family and his concerns about school. He had taught Tom to Indian wrestle and how to swing a baseball bat. When Tom became comfortable with the perpetrator's touch in sports, he allowed his friend to hug and fondle him. Then Tom was photographed nude in athletic poses. Finally the perpetrator made manual/genital contact and ultimately took pornographic photos. In foster care, Tom's foster parents were perplexed about the anxiety and acting out Tom displayed when they tried such routine activities to enhance Tom's self-esteem as teaching him sports, giving him small jobs, hugging him, or telling him he looked nice. They finally began to appreciate the complexity of Tom's situation when they were photographing him, and Tom asked if he was supposed to take his clothes off. With horror, they realized that each of their innocent attempts to build self-esteem had been perceived by Tom as a prolonged seduction attempt, replicating his earlier experience.

INFORMATION NEEDED

Foster parents need full information about the sexual abuse incident and the progression of events which were part of the seduction including nonsexual ways in which the perpetrator gained the child's trust or cooperation to avoid inadvertent replication of the child's earlier experiences. It is important for foster parents to be aware of the context of the incidents. Where did the sexual abuse take place? What time of day was it? If the location of the episodes is not known, foster parents should be informed that the three most likely places for the sexual abuse to have occurred are bathroom, bedroom, and car. With this understanding, foster parents can be careful not to be alone with children in these settings.

The agency has a legal responsibility to provide foster parents with the information relevant to the care of the child (Hardin & Tazzara, 1983). Failure to do so can result in situations which jeopardize the safety of both foster parents and child. Many of the false allegations of sexual abuse lodged against foster parents involve the child's misinterpretation of foster parent behavior, because the child perceives the situation to be similar to a former experience (McFadden & Stovall, 1984). Many substantiated allegations involve younger children who had been sexually abused prior to placement and acted out with sexualized behaviors which were misperceived as sexual cues (McFadden & Ryan, 1986). An agency which avoids fully informing foster parents in order to protect them from the reality of the child's past risks setting up the foster parents and an ultimate liability situation:

Cindy, age four, was placed in a foster home because she had been sexually abused by her stepfather. The agency did not inform the foster parents of any of the particulars, nor did they make it clear that Cindy was a sexually abused child. The context of Cindy's earlier sexual abuse was that in the evening, after Cindy's mother left for work, her stepfather took Cindy into the bathroom, undressed her, fondled her, then exposed himself and had Cindy touch his penis while he helped and masturbated to orgasm. Cindy had learned what was expected of her. One night in the foster home, the foster mother began to bathe Cindy, then realized she was late to a PTA meeting. She asked her husband to come in and finish the bath. Soon Cindy was alone in the bathroom with the new daddy. Her new mother had left. Cindy was naked. The new daddy rubbed her dry with a towel, which seemed to Cindy like the way her other daddy used to touch her. Believing that she knew what was expected of her, Cindy reached out to touch her new daddy's penis and try to unzip his pants.

In this incident the foster father did not respond to Cindy's overture. He called a neighbor for help so that Cindy could be dressed and put to bed by a female. The lack of information, however, led the foster family to inadvertently create a situation in which Cindy believed she should act sexually. Although Cindy's foster father did not respond, it is important to realize that some foster parents, feeling under stress, emotionally deprived, or curious might react differently to the child's cues. The child is not hoping for sexual activity but is misreading a situation based on earlier experience and is behaving in a way which he or she believes will please the adult. The foster parents need full information about the child's sexual abuse history including the child's relationship with the perpetrator, how the perpetrator gained compliance, progression of events leading up to the incident, the time of day it occurred, the location, and the child's earlier experience with family life in general. This will include the child's role in the family, relationship with both parents and siblings, the family's general communication system, family communication about sexuality, and how the child got needs met in the family. Foster parents should also be familiar with the child's vocabulary about body parts and sexuality.

Foster parents need to be advised that boys often do not report sexual abuse. Boys have difficulty in acknowledging sexual abuse because of the conflicting expectation of male sex roles (Nasjleti, 1980). Many boys are fearful that sexual abuse will make them less male because boys are not supposed to be victims. They also have grave concerns that an incident of sexual abuse with a male perpetrator means that they are gay.

Their reaction is further complicated by the fact that many boys experience erections during a sexual abuse episode and fear that this means that they wanted the abuse. Boys need both education and reassurance that an erection can be an involuntary response (like a sneeze) and doesn't necessarily mean purposeful enjoyment, that their gender identity was established when they were quite young and the incident did not change them to girls, and that sexual orientation does not depend on a single incident or series of incidents but on complex factors over an extended period of time. If they perceived themselves as heterosexuals and felt like heterosexuals prior to the incident then that is still their orientation. It is likely that there are many male children and youth in care who have been sexually abused and have never discussed it or come to terms with it.

The treatment team, including specialized foster parents, should be familiar with the indicators of sexual abuse in male children as well as females. Boys who have been anally penetrated often have difficulties with fecal impaction, fecal retention, diarrhea, spastic colon or constipation as a somatization of the tension and anxiety surrounding the incident. Boys who have been orally penetrated may exhibit gagging, spitting, vomiting, nausea, and digestive upsets. Foster parents report that children, boys and girls, who were victims of forced oral sex have great difficulty in eating any foods which may resemble ejaculate. They may refuse or become ill when served vanilla ice cream, tapioca, or cream of wheat.

Sexually abused boys may act out aggressively, either exploring with younger children or physically fighting when another person gets too close. They may want to enroll in martial arts and display a strong interest in self-protection. Often sexually abused boys display a certain subtle stiffness or tension between the waist and the knees, as if sensation was blocked and the body kept rigid. They don't like people coming up behind them. Wetting and soiling appear fairly frequently in sexually abused boys, although both can be tied to a number of other issues in the development of a child. Nighttime accidents appear to be linked to the disturbing nightmares and restless sleep that are common among sexual abuse victims. Some daytime wetting and soiling appears to be related to the child's dissociation from body sensation which may serve as a defense against the physical or psychological trauma of the incident.

Foster parents are to be trained as part of the therapeutic team to recognize indicators of possible sexual abuse and to contact the worker and therapist when the possibility of sexual abuse has been raised. Boys often find their way into specialized foster care for reasons of aggressive acting out, emotional disturbance or developmental lag without having been accurately diagnosed regarding their sexual abuse victimization. Therapeutic intervention can not only help the youth, it can also decrease the possibility of the intergenerational repetition of the pattern of molestation.

BEHAVIORS OF THE SEXUALLY ABUSED CHILD

Each child who has been sexually abused is first and foremost a child with all the normal needs of children. All children need attention, affection, and feeling of being loved and special to someone. All children need to feel good about themselves and to feel safe and good in their bodies. All children need a degree of freedom to explore their world, and all children need to have some limits set for them. Children who have been sexually abused are more like other children than different. Foster parents of sexually abused children require an educational grounding in the normal development of children. They especially need to know about the normal sexual development of children so they do not mistake normal behaviors such as masturbation and self-exploration as signs of sexual abuse (Chiaro, Marden et al., 1982).

The foster parent's task in managing the behaviors of the sexually abused child must be based on understanding of what the behavior is all about and the knowledge that the behavior may be a form of communication about the earlier sexual abuse. In addition to the normal tasks of parenting such as modeling appropriate behavior, explaining rules, setting limits and providing positive and negative consequences, the foster parents role is also one of teaching the child (Ryan, 1983). Foster parents, as part of the therapeutic team, need to understand why certain forms of punishment are prohibited by agency policy and why they would be damaging to children who have been sexually abused.

Spanking is never acceptable with children who have been sexually abused. It involves the foster parent touching the private parts of the child without the child's permission and undermines everything the therapeutic team is trying to teach the child about body integrity. It involves force. For some children it may be sexually stimulating. Similarly the old-fashioned technique of washing a child's mouth out with soap should be prohibited. For children who have had oral genital contact it recapitulates the experience of having something aversive forced into the mouth. Foster parents are able to discard punitive techniques (McFadden & Ryan, 1986) and focus on helping the child grow emotionally and learn new skills as they understand discipline as a teaching role.

The social worker may use inappropriate touching by the foster child to help foster parents consider questions such as the following: Why might a child touch others inappropriately? What does it mean to the foster family? Why might it bother them? What are the long-range consequences of the behavior? Foster parents have a variety of options to consider for dealing with inappropriate touching. They can avoid situations in which the child touches inappropriately; the child may sit next to Daddy to read a story rather than sit on his lap, or the child can be given a stuffed toy to hold and touch. A clear explanation must be given to the child:

> I understand that you are trying to be nice to me, but in our family and most families, we don't touch people there or in that way. We can give each other hugs, if we ask, or we can shake hands, like this.

When sexually abused children touch inappropriately, they may be feeling emotionally needy and are reverting back to a method they used in the past as a means of obtaining attention or affection. The treatment team needs to explore ways to provide an appropriate antidote to the child's underlying emotional neglect. Foster parents will be pleased and relieved to discover that when they focus on the child's emotional neglect and work to make the child feel secure, many of the difficult behaviors will fade away (McFadden, 1986).

Other behaviors of sexually abused children which concern foster parents include excessive or public masturbation, foul language, sexually aggressive play with younger children, seductive clothing or inappropriate exposure of the body, and wetting or soiling. The treatment team needs to sort out whether the behavior is an attempt to communicate about the sexual abuse, a bid for affection or attempt to please the foster parent, or outside of a child's conscious control. Social workers and therapists must understand the potency of these behaviors for provoking abuse and place top priority in supporting the foster parent to change the behavior. "Just ignore the behavior, it will go away" is poor advice which leads to further harm to the child.

PROTECTING THE CHILD
WHO HAS BEEN SEXUALLY ABUSED

Workers and foster parents need to be aware that a child's development tends to be arrested at the time of trauma and that sexually abused children may have developmental lag. Additionally they display behaviors which may make them vulnerable to further exploitation. Close monitoring and supervision is necessary during the time that the child is healing. Workers should be in frequent contact with the foster home and use visits as an opportunity to monitor the interaction between the child and the foster family. An indicator of potential revictimization is when the child becomes overly aligned with one foster parent, driving a wedge between the marital pair, and distancing the excluded spouse. Unrelated children are not necessarily included in an incest taboo protecting biological members (McFadden & Stovall, 1984). There can be more sexual activity between children in the home than workers wish to believe. Observation of the interactions of the sexually abused child with all family members is necessary to detect early signals of inappropriate sexual involvement between the foster child and any family member.

Foster parents need to be attuned to a child's potential for revictimization and to provide training and supervision to prevent that possibility. They must consider the developmental stage, not just chronological age, when they teach children responsibility for personal safety (Comfort, 1985). Situations which may seem safe for one's own nine-year old, such as walking home from school, may not be safe for a sexually abused child who has not learned the normal rules of self-protection. Other situations such as spending the night with an older friend or going camping should be examined carefully for potential risk. Children who have been sexually abused should not be left with adolescent baby-sitters who may not have the ego strengths to resist the child's cues. They probably need closer supervision when playing with other children. The agency should provide personal safety, sexual abuse prevention education for all children in care, and foster parents should reinforce the concepts of protection such as the child's right to say no in their dealings with children in the foster home. Foster parents may need to be reminded when children and youth are functioning at a developmental level below their chronological age to provide greater limits and supervision to protect the child.

PROTECTING THE FOSTER FAMILY

Foster parents must examine the rules, routines, and expectations of their home to successfully foster children who have been sexually abused. Innocent family activities which were a part of normal living with their own biological children can take on a confusing meaning to the foster child who doesn't know how to interpret the nonsexual intimacy of family living. Foster parents' own children may enjoy crawling under the covers in the parental bed or wrestling on the floor with a parent or older sibling. But such physical touching can take on a sexualized meaning to the child who has been sexually abused. Foster parents must reevaluate family activities through the eyes of a sexually abused child, decide which activities must be changed, and which rules must be enforced so that the foster child does not distort or misinterpret family touching. Guidelines for developing clear boundaries and reducing the possibility of confusion might include the following:

- Foster children of any age should not be allowed to get into bed with the foster parents. The foster parents' bedroom should be off-limits.
- No one touches another person without permission.
- Touching games such as tickling and wrestling should be prohibited as they involve touching without permission and may be uncomfortable or humiliating for the weaker child.
- All individuals old enough to care for themselves should have privacy for bathing, toileting, and dressing.
- A child who has been behaving seductively should not be alone with one other person.
- No one in the family should be outside the bedroom or bath-

room in underwear or pajamas without a bathrobe. Skimpy clothes should be restricted to pool or beach.
- Suggestive or obscene language is inappropriate. Children should be taught appropriate terminology for body parts.

One of the most important safeguards is for foster parents to set aside time for all children to communicate with them. They need to be especially aware that their own children could be at risk and inform their children explicitly to share with them any stories or activities engaged with the foster children. A no secrets rule is important. Foster parents' own children, regardless of age, should be given a simple explanation, geared to their level of cognition, that children coming into the home may have been sexually abused and might try some sexual activities with the other children. The natural children of foster parents should be included in the sexual abuse prevention training provided for the foster children or should have their own group.

FOSTER PARENTS' THERAPEUTIC ROLE

Regardless of how effective the clinical therapist may be in helping the child to come to terms with the sexual abuse and earlier emotional neglect the child still needs an important piece of therapy which only the foster home can provide. It is only through living in the family that the child unlearns the destructive messages of his earlier life and begins to grasp how a healthier family can operate. Some of the new messages the child will internalize through living in a specialized foster home are the following:

—Adults meet their needs with other adults, not with children.
—Adults do not use children to meet their needs.
—Children can be children, not substitute adults.
—We can all get our needs met and can ask for what we need.
—No one in the family uses force or bribery to get children to do things.
—Adults take care of children. Children do not have to take care of adults.

— No one child is the favorite or special one. All children are important. No child has to hold the family together.
— Everyone's feelings count. It's okay to talk about feelings.
— Sexuality is okay. It is different for adults and children.
— Some behaviors are appropriate in private but not in public.

Parents will help a child with remedial sex education in addition to modeling and explaining about family living. Many sexually abused children have precocious sexual knowledge beyond their years but lack the basics of sex education (Damon, Todd & Mc-Farlane, 1987). A child who swallowed semen, for example, may fear for years that a baby will start to grow in her stomach, or that she has somehow become rotten inside. Foster parents can help the child overcome anxieties and misconceptions by having sex education literature available appropriate for all ages and stages of development.

Children in therapy are able to handle and process the sexual abuse issues only at their current intellectual level of functioning. They may need to return to therapy as they grow older to deal with the anxieties generated by a new stage of development or to better lay to rest what happened in the past:

> A twelve-year-old female child had been in intensive therapy at age nine to help her deal with sexual abuse. By age ten and a half, her therapy seemed completed, and she began to grow and develop. At age twelve, at the onset of her menses, she stopped eating, had difficulty sleeping, and began leaving her soiled sanitary pads lying out in public view. The shift to a new developmental stage reactivated unresolved anxieties from her girlhood. She believed that the menstruation was proof that she had been terribly damaged inside by the penetration. Unable to verbalize this terrifying preoccupation, she attempted to get her foster parents to notice her bloody pads and respond to her fear.

Foster parents need to understand that therapy may be needed from time to time over the years and that a return to more intense treatment does not signify a failure on their part. Foster parents need to clarify with the therapist their current roles and the focus of treatment each time a child returns to therapy or enters a new phase of treatment. If the therapist is working with the child to promote self-esteem, the foster parent will be asked to perform adjunct activities to enhance the therapist's work. If the therapist is assisting the child in uncovering painful memories, the foster parents need anticipatory guidance in expecting some regression or sexual acting out and help to be able to provide a sheltering environment while the child is particularly fragile.

Children who have been sexually abused present many challenges to the specialized foster care agency. They bring with them many behaviors which can confound even the most experienced foster parents. Yet they are capable of growth and recovery if the emotional neglect which underlay the sexual abuse is addressed and the focus is not narrowly on controlling the sexualized behaviors. A teamwork relationship is required to reduce the risk of further exploitation for these vulnerable children. It is equally imperative to foster parents to have information about normal child development and fostering sexually abused children, and to reinforce this knowledge with close social work supervision. When the foster parents, worker, and therapist mutually understand the child and share common treatment goals, the child's emotional needs will be met, and he or she will be ready to learn new and positive messages about family living.

Chapter 8

Foster Parents of Mentally Retarded and Physically Handicapped Children

Susan Whitelaw Downs

ABSTRACT. Two surveys of foster parents find substantial numbers of current foster parents receptive to the idea of offering care to mentally retarded or physically handicapped children although the extent of the child's disability is a factor in the decision. Barriers to providing care to such children include maternal employment outside the home, foster parents' concerns about the demands that would be made on them, and their ability to cope. Foster parents appear to find agency services regarding foster care of disabled children adequate although the level of reimbursement may be too low to cover the costs of care and may negatively affect retention of experienced foster parents.

An important concern of child welfare professionals in the 1980s is the use of foster family care to meet the needs of children with developmental disabilities. Until about twenty years ago, such children were often considered unsuitable for foster family care and were placed in institutions if unable to remain with their families. With the deinstitutionalization movement of the late 1960s, however, agencies have made efforts to adapt foster family care programs to accommodate children with special characteristics. Partic-

Susan Whitelaw Downs is Assistant Professor at the School of Social Work, Wayne State University, 201 Cohn Building, 5557 Cass Avenue, Detroit, MI 48202.

The author wishes to thank Laura Howard, MSW, for research assistance in preparing this article.

ularly important in this adaptation process is the reconceptualization of the foster parents' role. As foster parents are increasingly expected to participate as part of the treatment team on behalf of the special needs children placed in their home, their role is becoming more professionalized. Good parenting skills are still necessary, as with regular foster care, but in addition foster parents may need to be recruited and trained with a focus on the demands of their role in treatment.

The research presented here addresses questions important to agencies working with foster parents and children with developmental disabilities.[1] The research reports results of two surveys of foster parents, including those fostering mentally retarded children and children with physical handicaps. For these foster parents, the research addresses such questions as the following: What are the characteristics of foster parents interested in caring for developmentally disabled children? What are the concerns foster parents have in deciding whether or not to provide care for developmentally disabled children? Do foster parents perceive agency services to be adequate in assisting them to provide foster care to children with developmental disabilities? Does a relationship exist between the foster parents' assessment of the adequacy of agency services and their willingness to continue offering foster care to children with developmental disabilities? Information on these questions could help agencies in recruiting, retaining, and supporting foster parents of mentally retarded or physically handicapped children.

CHILDREN WITH DEVELOPMENTAL DISABILITIES AND SOCIAL WORK

Historically, social workers as a group have not been heavily involved in the fields of mental retardation and developmental disabilities (Horejsi, 1979). Since the late 1960s, however, due in part to the deinstitutionalization movement, social workers have become

---

1. In this study, the term "developmental disability" is used to describe children who, according to their foster parents, are mentally retarded or physically handicapped. The extent to which these children meet the definition in the Developmental Disability Act (p.L. 95-602-1981) is not known.

actively involved in the development of community-based programs for the developmentally disabled (DeWeaver, 1983). The increase in the use of foster family care for developmentally disabled children is one manifestation of the trend to retain these children in the community (Appathurai et al., 1986; Arcari & Betman, 1986; Davis et al., 1984). Several programs and agencies in the United States are demonstrating that seriously handicapped children can be successfully maintained in foster family care (Tremitiere, 1979; Stepleton, 1987; Foster & Whitmore, 1986).

The public child welfare sector is also experiencing an increase in the proportion of foster children it serves who have special needs. It is estimated that about 22 percent of the foster children served by public child welfare agencies in 1983 had one or more disabling conditions (Tatara & Pettiford, 1985, p.68).

The trend toward placing children in foster care rather than institutions dovetails with another trend in child welfare, the professionalization of the foster parents' role. This trend is particularly important in considering quality of care for developmentally disabled children, since the foster parents are the primary providers of treatment programs designed to maximize the child's potential for growth (Galaway, 1978; Coyne, 1986; Tinney, 1985).

DATA SOURCES

The major source of data for the research reported here is the 1980 Survey of Foster Parents in Eight States, conducted by Westat, Inc. and the eight state child welfare agencies involved, with support from the U.S. Children's Bureau. The eight states are Arkansas, Alabama, Virginia, North Dakota, Utah, Rhode Island, Wisconsin, and Texas. A random sample of about 200 foster parents per state was drawn from state universe lists of licensed foster parents. The response rate was 79 percent. The present study uses a subsample of foster parents (n = 874) from the survey who were providing regular foster care (those providing group home care, emergency care, or preadoptive homes were excluded).

This study also used data from a survey of foster parents affiliated with two child welfare agencies in Detroit, Michigan.[2] These data were collected in 1986 with a sample of 200 foster parents. The survey questionnaire was based on the 1980 survey, with additional questions regarding financial aspects of foster care. In this report, all statistics are from the 1980 survey unless the 1986 survey is specifically indicated.

THE FOSTER FAMILIES

This portion of the analysis concerns the extent of interest among public agency foster parents in fostering developmentally disabled children, and the characteristics of those interested in doing so. The foster parents in the 1980 survey were asked if they were interested in caring for a mentally retarded or physically handicapped child. Regarding mentally retarded children, 39 percent of the foster parents said that they would probably accept such a child, 36 percent would possibly accept such a child, depending on the extent of the disability, and 26 percent said that they would probably not accept such a child. In all, 536 foster parents, or 75 percent of those surveyed, said that they were interested in fostering a mentally retarded child (probably or possibly would accept such a child).

Regarding physically handicapped children, the corresponding percentages indicate that 47 percent probably would accept, 27 percent possibly would accept, depending on the extent of the disability, and 27 percent probably would not accept. 633 foster parents (72 percent of those surveyed) were probably or possibly interested in caring for a physically handicapped child.

Table 1 displays characteristics of foster parents interested in caring for (probably or possibly would accept) a mentally retarded or physically handicapped child. Looking at the two groups together, the table shows that the foster parents interested in caring for either type of child tended to be experienced at fostering. Nearly half had

2. The two agencies cooperating in this survey were Children's Aid Society and Judson Center. The author thanks Dr. Bennie Stovall and Ms. Dorothy Mardeusz and other staff of these agencies for making the study possible. Funding for The Detroit Survey came from the Center for Urban Studies, the School of Social Work and Wayne State University, and Children's Aid Society.

Table 1: Characteristics of Foster Parents Interested in Caring for a
Mentally Retarded or Physically Handicapped Child (1986 survey)

Foster Parent Characteristic	Mentally Retarded Child (percents)	Physically Handicapped Child (percents)
Years a foster parent		
Less than one year	13	14
One to five years	40	41
Over five years	47	45
Total number of foster children cared for		
0 to 5	42	43
6 to 10	21	23
11 or more	37	34
Marital Status		
Married	83	86
Single	17	14
Annual Income		
Less than $7000	16	12
$7000 to less than $15000	34	35
$15000 to less than $25000	36	37
$25000 or more	14	17
Foster mother employment		
Working full time	15	18
Working part-time	14	14
Full time homemaker	71	68
Foster mother education		
8th grade or less	14	11
Some high school	24	21
High school graduate	54	57
Some college or college graduate	8	11
Foster mother age		
18 to 25	3	4
26 to 40	44	47
41 to 60	42	41
61 or older	11	8
Ethnicity		
Black	28	23
White	67	71
Hispanic, Native American, Asian	5	6
Total number of foster parents intrested in caring for this type of child	536	633

fostered over five years, and over half had cared for at least six foster children in the past. Over 80 percent were married. About half had annual incomes under $15,000 in 1980. Over two thirds of the foster mothers had graduated from high school, though few had continued their education past graduation. About half of the foster mothers were under age 40. About a quarter of the foster parents interested in caring for a developmentally disabled child were Black, about 5 percent were Hispanic, Native American, or Asian, and the rest were White.

For each type of disability (mental retardation or physical handicap) a comparison was made between those interested in fostering such a child (probably or possibly would accept) and those who were not (probably would not accept). Regarding mentally retarded children, those interested in caring for these children tended to have fostered more children than had those who were not interested in caring for such a child (chi square = 13.29, df = 2, p = .001). They were likely to have somewhat lower incomes (chi square = 12.96, df = 3, p = .004). In other respects, those interested in caring for mentally retarded children were similar to other foster parents in the survey.

A comparison of those interested in caring for a physically handicapped child with those who were not revealed the following differences in these two groups. Foster families interested in caring for a physically handicapped child were likely to have fostered more children (chi square = 10.808, df = 2, p = .01); the foster mothers were more likely to be married (chi square = 3.98, df = 1, p = .05); to be full-time homemakers (chi square = 5.71, df = 2, p = .05); to have more years of education (chi square = 2.17, df = 3, p = .05); and to be younger (chi square = 13.85, df = 3, p = 000). In other characteristics measured, those interested in caring for physically handicapped children were not significantly different from those who would probably not accept such a child.

All those foster parents surveyed were asked an open-ended question on what would be their major concerns in caring for a developmentally disabled child. Answers to this question indicate that the major concern of foster parents was the special demands made on them and their ability to cope with a child of this type. Very few foster parents mentioned such concerns as space in the home or acceptance of the child in the community as factors in deciding whether or not to care for a disabled child.

The following conclusions seem reasonable regarding the interest of public agency foster parents in caring for developmentally disabled children. First, a substantial proportion of these foster parents are receptive to the possibility of caring for such children, though the extent of the child's disability and the additional demands anticipated on the foster parents' time and coping ability are important considerations in their decision. A second and related conclusion is that outside employment limits the foster mother's willingness to care for a disabled child. Third, lower levels of education are associated with interest in caring for a mentally retarded child, while higher levels of education are associated with interest in caring for the physically handicapped. The implications of this finding for the quality of fostering provided to developmentally disabled children are not known.

FOSTERING MENTALLY RETARDED CHILDREN

Foster parents with experience in caring for mentally retarded foster children were asked questions about the adequacy of agency services while they were caring for this type of child. Two aspects of the agency services were included in the 1980 survey: information on the child's background and special needs, and help and support in dealing with the child's special needs or problems. A question on the adequacy of payments to cover the costs of care was included on the 1986 survey. (See Table 2.) Overall, thirty-one percent of the foster parents surveyed had had experience in caring for a mentally retarded child (n = 268). About 70 percent of these experienced foster parents said that they had received adequate information about the child's background and special needs from the agency. About 80 percent of these foster parents said that they received adequate help and support from the agency in dealing with the child's special needs or problems during the time that they cared for a mentally retarded child.

Foster parents in the 1980 survey conducted in eight states were not asked about the adequacy of board rates for foster children. However, the Detroit survey did address this issue. About 69 per-

Table 2:   Adequacy of agency services to foster parents of
developmentally disabled children.

Service	Mentally Retarded Child (percents)	Physically Handicapped Child (percents)
Information on child's background or special needs		
adequate	70	79
not adequate	30	21
Help or support in dealing with the child's special needs or problems		
adequate	80	84
not adequate	20	16
*Data Source: 1980 suvey		
N	268	237

Payments to cover the costs of care		
adequate	69	54
not adequate	31	46
Data Source: 1986 survey		
N	22	35

cent of the Detroit foster parents with experience in caring for mentally retarded children stated that they found the board rate adequate to cover expenses. Daily payment rates for regular foster care in Michigan in 1986 were $10.10 for age 0-12 and $12.50 for age 13-18.

It was of interest to discover whether a relationship existed between the foster parents' assessment of the adequacy of agency services they received while caring for a mentally retarded child and their willingness to offer foster care to other mentally retarded children. A bivariate analysis was conducted comparing foster parent's assessment of the adequacy of agency services with whether or not they were willing to foster another mentally retarded child. Table 3 shows the results of the bivariate analysis. Overall, about 81 percent of the experienced foster parents said that they were willing to care for another mentally retarded child, while 19 percent were unwilling to continue to offer this type of care. As Table 3 shows, 71 percent of those willing to continue said that the information they received from the agency on the child's background was adequate, whereas 62 percent of those unwilling to continue found this area of agency service to be adequate. Eighty percent of those planning to continue fostering mentally retarded children believed that the help they received from the agency in dealing with the child's special

Table 3: Foster parent assessment of adequacy of agency services by willingness to care for another mentally retarded child

Agency Service for previous MR child	Willing to Foster Another MR Child	
	Yes (%)	No (%)
Information on child's background or special needs*		
adequate	71	62
not adequate	29	38
Help or support in dealing with the child's special needs or problems*		
adequate	80	76
not adequate	20	24
*Data Source: 1980 Survey		
N	218	50
Percent	81	19
Payments to cover costs of care**		
adequate	76	50
not adequate	24	50
**Data Source: 1986 Survey		
N	21	8
Percent	72	28

Note: The question on the adequacy of payments was not asked on the 1980 Survey, but was asked on the 1986 Survey.

needs or problems was adequate; 76 percent of those not planning to continue found this area of agency service to be adequate. The Detroit survey shows that 76 percent of the foster parents who were willing to continue found the payments adequate to cover the costs of care, while only 50 percent of those unwilling to continue found the payments sufficient to cover the cost of care.

FOSTERING PHYSICALLY HANDICAPPED CHILDREN

Regarding the foster parents of physically handicapped children, the study found that 27 percent of the foster parents in the 1980 survey (N = 237) had had experience in caring for such a child. (See Table 2.) Seventy-nine percent of the foster parents found information on the physically handicapped child's background and special needs to be adequate. Eighty-four percent found the help and support received from the agency regarding the child's problem or special needs to be adequate. Fifty-four percent found payments to cover the cost of care to be adequate (1986 survey).

Table 4 summarizes the results of a bivariate analysis on perception of adequacy of agency services to willingness to foster another physically handicapped child.

IMPLICATIONS FOR AGENCY PRACTICE

The findings of this study have implications for the recruitment and provision of services to foster parents for developmentally disabled children.

Recruitment

The results of these analyses indicate that a fairly large percentage of current foster parents would be interested in fostering a child with developmental disabilities. This suggests that resources do exist for the growing number of developmentally disabled children requiring foster care placement in the public child welfare sector.

The finding that those women interested in fostering disabled children were less likely than other foster mothers to be working outside the home may mean that foster parent supply for disabled

Table 4: Foster parent assessment of adequacy of agency services by
willingness to care for another physically handicapped foster child.

Agency service for previous PH child	Willing to Foster Another PH Child	
	Yes	No
	(%)	(%)
Information on child's background or special needs*		
adequate	79	77
not adequate	21	23
Help or support in dealing with the child's special needs or problems*		
adequate	85	77
not adequate	15	23
*Data Source: 1980 Survey		
N	203	30
Percent	87	13
Payments to cover costs of care**		
adequate	59	33
not adequate	41	67
**Data Source: 1986 Survey		
N	22	6
Percent	79	21

Note: The question on the adequacy of payments was not asked on the
1980 Survey, but was asked on the 1986 Survey.

children will depend, in part, on labor market opportunities for
women. Other research on foster parent supply supports the finding
of the present report that labor market employment decreases the
amount of foster care that foster parents can provide (Campbell and
Downs, 1987). The extent to which higher reimbursement rates for
fostering disabled children would attract women to fostering and
away from market employment is not known but deserves study.

Foster parents, in considering fostering a developmentally disabled child, expressed concern about the demands such care would
make on them. Also, they take into account the extent of the child's
disability. This suggests that recruitment efforts should include concrete information on the expectations made on foster parents for this

type of care and on the characteristics of the children. In order for foster parents to make an informed judgment on whether or not they would be suitable as care-givers for disabled children, they need to know what kind of care the child needs, what the demands will be on the family, and what kind of special information or training will be needed. This finding supports the view of McFadden (1985) that experienced foster parents are effective recruiters and trainers of new foster families, since they have the necessary information from firsthand experience.

Payment Levels

The study found that level of payments may be the most problematic of the services that agencies provide to foster parents. A substantial minority of the Detroit foster parents surveyed found that payment levels were inadequate to cover the costs of caring for a mentally retarded or physically handicapped child. The findings offer limited support to the view that foster parents who find payments inadequate are somewhat less willing than others to continue offering care for developmentally disabled children. This conclusion is offered cautiously, since the relationship of perceived adequacy of payment to willingness to continue is not statistically significant at the .05 level or less. However, these findings do support previous research indicating that payment levels in foster care are insufficient to cover the costs that foster parents incur (DeJong, 1975; Specht, 1975; Settles et al., 1976) and that low levels of reimbursement negatively affect the amount of foster care families are able to provide (Simon, 1975; Campbell and Downs, 1987; Downs, 1989). Further research is needed to clarify whether increasing foster care payment rates for children with developmental disabilities would enhance retention of these foster parents.

Regarding other kinds of agency services, the study suggests that overall foster parents find adequate the information and casework support they receive from the agency regarding children in their care. Also, the study found only very limited support for the view that the level of adequacy of information provided and casework support will positively affect retention of foster parents. The results show that foster parents who were willing to continue fostering disabled children were only slightly more likely to have found agency services adequate than did those who were not planning to continue, and overall the differences were small and did not attain statistical significance. Clearly, factors outside the agency's control will affect retention, such as foster parents' age or other life circumstances. Still, common sense and other research suggests that foster parents who feel well supported by the agency are likely to continue fostering longer than those who do not feel well supported (Cautley, 1980; Boyd & Remy, 1979).

In summary, this study found that a substantial number of current foster parents, licensed by public child welfare agencies, are receptive to the idea of offering care to mentally retarded or physically handicapped children, though the extent of the child's disability is a factor in the decision. Barriers to providing care to such children include maternal employment outside the home, foster parents' concern about the demands that would be made on them, and their ability to cope. In general, the majority of foster parents appear to find agency services regarding the foster care of disabled children to be adequate, though level of reimbursement rates may be too low to cover the costs of care and may negatively affect retention of foster parents experienced in this type of care.

Chapter 9

Treatment Foster Home Care
for Autistic Children

Clarice E. Rosen

ABSTRACT. A foster parent describes how therapeutic foster parents can provide autistic children with a consistent, structured, warm, nurturing, and supportive family atmosphere that stimulates growth. Autistic children are consistently taught the tasks and behaviors which are desired by breaking tasks down into small components and teaching on a step-by-step basis; gentle but consistent firmness is asserted to assure that the child follows through on the desired task. Consistency between the child's outside of home and inside of home experiences is essential. Thus foster parents work closely with schools, birth parents, and others who are in contact with the child to assure that the child is experiencing a consistent, nurturing environment.

I must have been very persuasive eighteen years ago when I talked a husband and five children into enlarging our family with more "knee huggers." Ignorant as we were about the challenges of foster care, we decided to do something about the call for foster homes and have a couple of "poster kids" living with us. We had a family of five children: four sons, and one daughter. The oldest son was just starting high school and our daughter, the youngest, was a preschooler. We liked challenges and we loved kids.

Our family eventually filled out to six boys and three girls, three of them very difficult autistic children and I was challenged from

Clarice E. Rosen is a Therapeutic Foster Home Parent affiliated with the Wilder Children's Placement Service, 565 Holly Avenue, St. Paul, MN 55102.

early morning to late at night and sometimes most of the night. Though that wasn't quite the challenge or the population our original wanting to help was meant to be, we were never sorry. Tired, certainly, but not sorry. The pain and guilt of separation we experienced when the first three autistic young adults were moved to group homes, was our biggest challenge.

We have no college degrees and when our first autistic child moved in, we knew zero about autism. Our experience and knowledge of child rearing comes initially from our own "home-made" family and their many playmates. Fifteen years ago libraries had little enlightening information to offer. Information on etiology, programs, and research was just beginning to be disseminated. The local chapter of the National Society for Autistic Children became a source for information and publications as well as a support group. Our home-made children and social workers contributed the publications they came across while we continued to search libraries and bookstores. We researched medical and psychological journals and attended workshops and lectures. My husband, Bob, calls himself "Assistant Director" while I am "Director," which is to say he is the chef and chief financial officer and I am the program director and teacher and all other tasks are shared. Originally I was the at-home parent but when Bob retired from his own business, we divided responsibilities according to our skills and interests.

HISTORY AND DEFINITION

Autism is a low-incident (5 out of every 10,000 births), lifelong disability. It is four times more common in males than females. The name is from the Greek word "autos" meaning self. Dr. Leo Kamner first described autism in 1943 and compiled a checklist of behaviors to be observed and used in the diagnosis. Observation in a variety of settings is the only tool for the diagnosis of autism. Professionals have been, and some may still be, reluctant to make the diagnosis of autism. It wasn't until the early 60s that doctors would recognize it as a separate phenomena from childhood schizophrenia.

Behavior and responses, severe or subtle, can be atypical from birth. Some of the early concerns reported by parents are the frequent episodes of screaming and crying, the child's rigidity when held or touched and fears that a child may be going deaf. Autistic children have unusual, abnormal, or bizarre reactions to what they see, hear and/or feel. Gait and body posture are often unusual and they have abnormal ways of relating to people, objects and events. They may have disturbed sleep patterns. They seem withdrawn, having a tuned-out look in their eyes and seem to look through rather than at you. Frequently, they do not use language as a useful means of communication, but are mute or echolalic. They can be preoccupied with self-stimulating and ritualistic behaviors, i.e., arm flapping, finger flicking, rocking, toe walking, spinning objects and pacing. They can be obsessed with rituals and sameness; for example, moving objects that are out of place and arranging toys in a specific order. They are experts at manipulating people and testing limits.

Autistic children can be very aggressive: biting, kicking and scratching; and/or have some form of mild to extreme self-injurious behaviors from head banging to chewing on themselves. These behaviors can be persistent and resistive to change and require consistent unique management and treatment. Autistic children are functionally retarded but development is frequently uneven with isolated areas of greater skill and abilities.

PHILOSOPHY

Our philosophy as therapeutic foster parents is to provide the children with a consistent, structured, warm, nurturing and supportive family atmosphere that stimulates growth and potential. Essential for growth is an environment that is respectful, sensitive, and safe; where the children are not judged but praised and encouraged for attempts and the smallest successes. The therapeutic milieu is programmed to encompass the whole day and address all domains of development and daily living. We teach as many functional skills as possible, such as communication, self care, practical and family living, and social and leisure skills, using natural and aversive consequences, behavior modification techniques and crisis prevention methods.

Dedication, commitment and resourcefulness are crucial for effectively working with these children, given the high demands and needs of the autistic child. Persons who are willing to set goals and limits with determination to follow through and also, who can be patient and flexible when necessary, can effectively foster autistic children. Working with autistic children/people is a demanding, frequently frustrating, and stressful task, but the needed everyday-all day discipline of intense intrusion will be rewarded. The reward may be as simple as the autistic child holding your hand, brushing his teeth, or holding his fork correctly.

The three autistic children came to use at different ages, functioning levels, and prognosis for development and achievement. We also have a foster daughter who has been with us since she was six who is emotionally disturbed, mentally retarded, and physically handicapped. These four foster children along with our five home-made children made for a fairly heterogeneous group. A year ago we accepted placement of another autistic child who will be thirteen this fall. With the type and number of foster children we have, it is necessary for us to work as a couple, but certainly our five home-made children have been an immense asset. Our children became our chief child care workers providing not only respite but a support staff for appropriate modeling and intervention when necessary. They helped to make many activities more manageable. Certainly, they gained knowledge and understanding of some handicapping conditions, but most importantly they learned compassion for the less able. It has been a unique and unusual education for them.

We continue to have our biological daughter at home to provide still-necessary respite and support. The children are less likely to act out with someone familiar. While taking care of yourself and your needs can easily be put on "hold," the result is burnout. It is essential to have some system for respite care otherwise you cannot continue to be effective. However, the risk with having built-in child and respite care givers is having too closed a community and not providing an opportunity for the children to learn to adjust to new people and situations.

JERRY

Jerry was our first autistic foster child. He had his fourth birthday shortly after being placed with us but was not toilet trained and had just learned to walk. Jerry was "different" from birth, was termed a failure-to-thrive baby until a hospital assessment diagnosed him as autistic. He was very small for his age, was virtually mute, except for saying his name, seldom slept through the night and had frequent tantrums daily. His tantrums usually included some self-injurious behavior – head banging, tearing at his face and pulling his hair while screaming and/or crying.

His favorite activities were spinning objects, flapping his arms, rocking and toe walking. Unlike most autistic children, he fortunately liked to be held and touched and he would occasionally initiate some physical interaction, though at times it was like the manipulation of an inanimate object. He therefore would work for social reinforcement. Between tantrums, he looked like a fairly happy boy who was appealing and charming to people, but the psychiatrist's prognosis wasn't very optimistic.

Relative to the syndrome he now has good receptive and fair expressive language skills (using mostly phrases), has some independent self care and daily living skills, and is cooperative and appropriate at most social activities and events. His leisure time is now appropriately filled when he is directed to an activity. Work performance, when the job fits his ability and skill level, is slow but steady.

The care givers at the facility where he now lives report their continued surprise at the number of tasks and the level of his performance. The assaultive and disruptive behaviors continue to be a problem, especially when staff are not very knowledgeable or well trained in autism.

MARY JO

Mary Jo was, by far, the most difficult and the lowest-functioning child to come to our home. She was unpredictable, uncooperative, destructive and assaultive. Her method of communication was sounds, gestures and one word: "no." Her motor skills were poor: she couldn't tie, button, zip, comb, brush, toilet or wash herself. She could feed herself but her table manners were unpleasant and she daily threw food and beverages at meal time. Her assaultive behavior included spitting, scratching, biting, kicking and pulling hair and when possible, she aimed for the face/head. When she slept, it was only for short periods of a few hours. Periodically she would have several days and nights of wetting herself and refusing to eat until she discovered we wouldn't make an issue of it, but rather ignored the behavior. Stripping off her clothes regardless of where she was, even on the school bus, was one of her more bizarre behaviors. She had strange body posture and contortions. She would hold her breath and extended her stomach. Her gait was very clumsy. She had skin and respiratory allergies that needed daily and seasonal attention. In her late adolescence, she began having seizures.

Mary Jo's assets were her pretty appearance, when not posturing, and her ability to give and receive affection. Though perhaps not always sincere, she could initiate and accept such a gesture. She has remained mute but uses sign language as an appropriate modality for communication. She has learned to be more cooperative and predictable through the stable environment we offered her. She learned more mannerly table behavior, and with prompts and supervision, to brush her teeth, comb her hair and shower. She will always need total around-the-clock care, supervision and a protected living situation. She lives in a group home for autistic adults, while Jerry is living in a larger facility waiting for an opening in a smaller group home.

THE TEACHING PROCESS

Autistic children have to be taught almost everything. They cannot process sensory stimulation as most people do. Most tasks need to be taught, one on one—what hand to use when picking up a fork, with which to eat even if they have established a dominant side, how to turn the pages of a magazine, how to unscrew the cap on a tube of toothpaste, how to rub their hands together to wash them, how to hold the soap in preparation for washing, how to turn a doorknob to open a door, etc. Imagine the number of steps it would take for these children to learn to make a bed, to shower or bathe, to cut up food, comb hair, put clothes on a hook, shake hands and answer "What is your name?" And how about buttoning, tying, how to wipe with toilet paper, raise shades, turn a light on and off, how to fold hands, how to skip, use scissors, hold a pencil or color crayon, point a finger and use a knife to butter bread or cut food?

Consider the number of tasks to be learned in a morning routine up to eating breakfast—getting out of bed at a signal or command, turning on and off lights, raising shades, toileting, washing hands and face, making the bed, taking off pajamas and hanging them up, pick out clothing, dressing and combing hair, and so on. Now take one of those tasks and break it down into steps in the form of task analysis. For example, making the bed or washing hands, which has 11 steps to it: 1. Turn on the water. 2. Wet hands. 3. Pick up the soap. 4. Rub soap over hands. 5. Put soap back. 6. Rub hands together. 7. Rinse hands under water. 8. Turn off the water. 9. Pick up the towel. 10. Dry hands on towel. 11. Hang up the towel. An additional step would be to learn which is the hot or cold faucet.

Next you need to be realistic about the capabilities of the child to learn the steps of a task and the tasks in the routine. Questions to pose before beginning are: Will they be skilled and independent or always need assistance, prompts and/or supervision? How will the limit of their abilities be determined? The time will come as you approach each new step in a task when it is apparent that the limit has been reached. It is important though to be optimistic about the child's potential to perform the task before beginning training. There is harm in not being optimistic enough if one doesn't reevaluate expectations during the training process. Training may stop too early with a different approach not tried or criteria set too low.

The tools for teaching are verbal, visual and/or physical hands-on manipulation. Each step learned is "shaped" towards the goal and initially must be rewarded. Perhaps the method of backward chaining would be more successful for certain tasks. When teaching tying laces, for example, for immediate rewardable success, you may have the child do the last step first—pulling the bow tight with your assistance. Food is a strong reinforcer and initially you may need to use foods for the teaching of new tasks but it should be paired with the social rewards/reinforcers as well, so that eventually it can be dropped as a reinforcer. Examples are, "Good working" with a hug, pat on the back or a tickle or whatever is especially pleasing to the child.

Knowing how resistant autistic children can be, their potential for uncooperative, acting out, assaultive or self-injurious behavior, you can ignore, use natural consequences or use aversive measures, but behavior must be under control to gain cooperation. The child may have to be conditioned to have quiet or folded hands in preparation for working on a task. A loud and commanding voice to get their attention is necessary at times because autistic children have selective hearing and are passive/aggressive. When giving an instruction you need to be prepared to make them follow it. The direction "Pick up your toys, it's time to eat" can send the child directly to the kitchen. They only reacted to "eat" and you have no choice but to take the child back to the toys, manipulating his hands to pick up and saying "you may eat when the toys are picked up." The child may have been confused or tried to avoid the task but this is not a time for the child to have a choice. Other situations will provide opportunities for "no."

INTEGRATING WITH THE COMMUNITY

We worked hard for our children to be as functional and independent as their abilities would allow them, but were they transferable — could they generalize using their skills effectively in other environments? To help the generalization of skills it was necessary for us to vary the settings where tasks were performed, even learned, as much as possible. Perhaps, it was having them make another bed in another bedroom, clean a different bathroom, or shovel the neighbor's sidewalk. To insure school demanded and taught the same tasks and vice versa meant daily logging and communication with the teachers. Still, it was surprising to us when we learned that only one of the children would routinely ask to be excluded from the lunch table at school when here they did not leave our table with an "Excuse, please." Though it wasn't a major issue, it was an indication of inconsistent expectations. The I.E.P. (individual education plan) should, of course, state the goals and objectives but they usually are too global and not specific enough, a fault of the instrument. Brushing teeth under "self care" will not tell anyone they are being taught to use right or left hand, and it may just be right hand in school and left at home.

Communication between the care givers is essential, for instance, home to school, teachers to their aides, and between parents, the home care givers and between biological parents. Though the parents of our children admittedly could not give daily around-the-clock care, they often continued to have some relationships with their child. Sometimes the contact was a visit of a few hours or a weekend at their home. Sometimes, to ensure it was a positive occurrence, and to support and model methods for dealing with behaviors, the visit was under our supervision.

Sometimes the parents' guilt and pain is overwhelming; perhaps the autistic child has been an issue in the discord or destruction of a marriage and family. However, for a more healthy prognosis, parent involvement and acceptance as part of the team is paramount. Only when the child has been placed in foster care at a very young age and there is no discernible attachment, does it seem less important for the child, but it usually is still an issue for the parent. Their capability to lend us, the foster parents, support is always important and it certainly helps to have an amicable relationship with the parents. They need to know about their child.

In spite of the stigma and less than positive image with which society has historically viewed foster care and in spite of the need to accept another set of parents for their child, the biological parents have been able to be a part of our foster children's care and treatment on some level if they desire it. Perhaps their main involvement can be as an advocate for their child in the community and who better, for frequently they are the ones most readily listened to.

It is always a better treatment plan to have consistency across all possible environments. Without this consistency, autistic children could regress and undo months of work and certainly hamper progress. Therefore we need to have a workable system of communication with parents, discussing methods for teaching or modifying behaviors and communicating their expectations and hope for their child's future. Agency quarterly staffings, schools' individual educational planning (IEP), regular phone conversations and dialogue before and after visits are the mechanisms for the exchange of ideas, concerns and methods.

It is rewarding for us to know the children can and will transfer some skills when on visits and to see the parents take some joy from their child's progress. We could share in the joy and pride of the child's accomplishments, laugh together over the amusing and sometimes bizarre escapades and even cry together over trials and hopeless dreams. The parents of our children are usually accepting of the continued need for out-of-home placement for their children so it is then necessary for all of us to have and agree on a plan for the future.

It may be easier for parents to support treatment foster care and see it as a permanent option over a residential facility. Foster homes offer stability that is not usually possible in a larger facility where staff turnover is frequent. This allows for parents to develop a relationship with the foster parent while providing a better environment for the child's development.

Once the autistic child is in the welfare system, they seem to stay in the system and so the optimal situation would be the availability of treatment foster homes for all autistic children. Without the continued support and involvement of the biological parent/parents, an already arduous job would be that much more difficult. While transition is always traumatic for autistic children/adults, it is much less so if they have a system for support and involvement from all the people who have cared for and about them.

COMMUNITY EDUCATION AND ADVOCACY

There are always issues that need to be addressed and advocated for autistic children, not only because of the size of the population affected but because their needs are so great. Programs are costly and without vigorous and assertive advocating, little attention would be given to existing or developing new programs for autistic children both in school and the community. Two of the issues are the fears and risks people associate with working with autistic children and the need to identify appropriate medical systems. Sitting in a doctor's crowded waiting room for a half hour for a routine physical or dental examination is a potentially difficult situation when the doctor is not willing or able to take the time our children require. Oftentimes these professionals do not have an adequate knowledge of autism. Nurses are sometimes better informed. Though children with autism can be appealing and charming, they are difficult and their issues equally so.

A question most often asked when addressing groups is "What are the effects of this foster child population on a foster family?" I can only answer that by pointing out how our home-made children continue to be interested—that they did not burn out! Through exposure to our interest in foster care and most specifically autistic children, they also developed and pursued similar interests. One son is a clinical psychologist; our daughter is about to graduate from college with a degree in psychology; another son is a foster parent, and another has been a Big Brother for another autistic child.

The drawbacks are that foster children require a lot of our time; the risk to everyone's physical safety; and people assuming we are a mental health facility and therefore that even our home-made children were handicapped. Laughter is not only healthy medicine but it eases stress and is helpful in hurdling the rough times. Sometimes it may sound close to hysteria but there is and was lots of laughter in our house.

In conclusion I will relate a story that will emphasize the types of behaviors possible from autistic children, the importance of humor, the need for dedication to foster parenting an autistic child, and what kinds of things you may be required to do.

It was one of the most memorable events in our house, a parting gift from Mary Jo and what Bob calls "The Chocolate Colored Morning."

I usually got Mary Jo up, but on this particular morning, I walked into her room, took one look and decided I could not handle what I saw alone. I didn't even know where to start! I went out in the hallway, breathed some fresh air and called Bob. Smiling, thinking it was something funny and ordinary like she probably stripped her pajamas off or had the pillow case over her head, he walked in and backed right out, gagging. Mary Jo had wet and soiled sometime during the night and "brown" was everywhere—on the walls, in her hair, ears, face, hands and feet and arms, and of course the bed clothing was covered!

When we had sufficiently composed ourselves, we decided on a course of action. Bob would move this tall, gangly, 17-year-old out of bed and get her into the shower, spreading the mess as little as possible and I would tackle the walls and bed. The blankets and sheets had to be hosed off outside first because my washing machine probably would have gone "absent without leave" otherwise.

Of course, as Mary Jo and bed clothing were removed, the "brown" was spread, in spite of efforts with plastic bags, pails of water and paper towels to confine the mess. At the time, we didn't view the event with much humor but the next day, when gagging had subsided, we could laugh about it. Mary Jo, of course, thought it was very funny from the start. This should convey why respite care is very necessary for the foster parent and why personal introspection is necessary when considering foster parenting an autistic child.

People have said to us they could not do it. They were probably right. It takes people who are resourceful, committed, realistic about their abilities, willing to put enormous amounts of effort into the job and willing to learn about autism and new ways of parenting. This is not for everyone and we have often felt alone, battered, bruised and discouraged but the rewards have always renewed our determination and dedication. We are hooked!

Chapter 10

Leaving Home Again:
Emancipation from Foster Family Care

Emily Jean McFadden
Dale Rice
Patricia Ryan
Bruce Warren

ABSTRACT. Young people emancipating from foster care are in the process of leaving home again. In addition to tangible independent living skills, these young people require assistance with the emotional, intangible aspects of emancipation including reliving the separation experience and confusion about their identity. Foster parents can be trained to assist youth in the emancipation process by understanding that preparation of the young person will often lead to a reactivation of earlier losses, maladaptive responses to separation and rejection, reunion fantasies, and may reactivate emotional scar tissue which has previously helped the young person with their loss experiences. Preparation of the young person for emancipation involves teamwork among social workers, therapists, and foster parents, as well as group experiences for the emancipating youth. Foster parents and youth may also be encouraged to maintain post-emancipation relationships.

Under the best of circumstances, emancipation can be a difficult process requiring a series of complex adaptations. A youth's ability

Emily Jean McFadden is Associate Professor, Social Work Department, Dale Rice is Professor in the Department of Special Education, Patricia Ryan is Administrative Director of the Institute for the Study of Children and Families, and Bruce Warren is Professor in the Department of Sociology, at Eastern Michigan University, Ypsilanti, MI 48197.

to adapt to new surroundings and greater independence is interactive with parental adjustments to their own new roles. The way various members of the family adapt and are able to move into new life stages is dependent on earlier family interactional patterns. For instance, if parents have used the child to stabilize a dysfunctional marital relationship, the youth will find leaving home very difficult.

There is a fine line between feeling free to go and feeling rejected. Many youth who seem eager to leave are ambivalent, and some don't want to go. Indeed many youth develop symptomatic behavior in order to avoid leaving home and the letting go process (Haley, 1980). This ambivalence is intensified for youth who have been in a series of out of home placements, which may have included family foster care, residential care, or failed adoptions. The leaving home process becomes problematic, compounded by a series of unresolved losses which resurface as the youth faces the uncertain future. Youth emancipating from their biological families are leaving home. Youth emancipating from foster care are leaving home *again*. They must deal with their sense of pain and rejection from earlier separations while confronting current losses.

Anderson and Simonitch (1981) describe the emancipation process among youth in foster care as one involving reactive depression:

> Letting go of a placement in a foster home or institution in which dependency needs are met and relationships are satisfying is difficult. Moving from one neighborhood to another, with the consequent loss of friends, complicates the problem. Most of these youths have had to break ties with their families of origin and have little if any family support to hold on to and buoy them up through the difficult life adjustment period. . . . Reactive depression of some degree is always a response to loss or disappointment. The reaction varies in intensity and duration, depending on the young person's personality strength, reconstitutive ability and capacity to compensate for losses and disappointments. (p. 385)

The young person in placement experiences a double loss. There is the real loss here and now: loss of security, home, relationships, neighborhood, and roles. Additionally the youth reexperiences, consciously or unconsciously, the loss of the biological family. For most children this may be experienced also as a loss of self. As the youth is poised for launching into the world, he or she relives the sum total of all prior losses including those engendered in prior placements.

The National Commission on Children in Need of Parents (1979) terms foster care "an unconscionable failure harming large numbers of the children it purports to serve" (p. 5). On the other hand, Jones and Moses (1984) found in a study of former foster children in West Virginia that the largest group of respondents were very satisfied with their foster care experience and over three quarters of the group expressed satisfaction. In a literature review of the impact of foster care on children, Maluccio and Fein (1985) found that with several exceptions, "researchers have consistently reported that foster care graduates function well and that no negative effect of foster care on the child's adjustment is detected" (p. 125). Festinger's (1983) study of former foster children found that on the whole the young adults were quite satisfied with their experience in foster care, and that "by and large those who felt their placement was necessary, and this was a large majority, expressed more satisfaction with their experience than those who felt they had been placed unnecessarily" (p. 257-259).

Fanshel and Shinn (1978) found caseworkers' ratings of children entering foster care provided little evidence of massive emotional trauma. Only a minority of the subjects displayed intense reactions to separation. They caution:

> We are not completely sure that continued tenure in foster care over extended periods of time is not in itself harmful to children. On the level at which we were able to measure the adjustment of the children we could find no such negative effect. However, we feel that our measures of adjustment are not without problems, and we are not sure that our procedures have captured the potential feelings of pain and impaired self-image that can be created by impermanent status in foster care. (p. 479)

CONCERNS OF YOUTH IN FOSTER CARE

Whatever the experiences of children leaving care, the plight of youth facing the transition to independent living has been amply documented (Barth, 1986; Cousins, 1983; Furrh, 1983; Griffin, 1985). As federal funds become available to develop training programs for emancipating youth and implementing emancipation services in the states, a variety of approaches and strategies have emerged. Many focus on teaching life skills (Euster, Ward, Varner and Euster, 1984), on developing transitional living arrangements (Furrh, 1983; Simonitch and Anderson, 1979), or increasing counseling services (Rowe, 1983). Typically, training programs focus on developing tangible skills such as caring for one's self, budgeting, finding employment or becoming an intelligent consumer. Less prevalent is a focus on the more intangible skills emancipating youth need in dealing with their feelings and developing appropriate interpersonal skills.

Young people in foster care are often silently preoccupied with problems and worries and may vigorously act out these feelings. Their behavioral messages baffle or provoke both foster parents and caseworkers. The primary message they are trying to communicate centers on the complex configuration of feelings about their families. These youth usually do not understand the reasons for their placement, or why they are separated from their families (Fanshel and Shinn, 1978; Horesji, 1979; Geiser, 1973). A study of former foster children found the following:

> In all cases a discrepancy was found between the subject's version and the agency's version of how the subject came into care, the core of which seemed to be the subject's need to perceive placement as an event forced upon child and parents by external society. Subjects were unable to perceive their parents as having personal failings preventing them from giving care to their children. (Rest and Watson, 1984, p. 298)

Frequently, even if the caseworker attempted to explain the reasons, the child was too distressed, too young, or simply unable to comprehend the events leading to separation. Such children may expend enormous emotional energy to preserve an idealized image of parents. Children reject explanations blaming their parents because they need to preserve a shaky sense of self. As they become adolescents they may be more able to understand their situation, if helped by their caseworker or therapist.

Young people in care typically suspect the separation occurred because they were bad, unworthy, or unlovable (Ryan, 1978; Geiser, 1973; Littner, 1956). This self-blame is reflected in diminished self-esteem. Gil and Bogart (1982) found that all foster children they studied scored somewhat lower than the standardized norm in self-esteem and that children in group homes scored even lower than children in family foster homes.

Lack of a clear identity is a major factor in poor self-esteem. Most children gain this identity from their family. The family is a mirror that reflects back who they are. However, for children in foster care, the original mirror is cracked or shattered. Multiple foster family placements become carnival fun house mirrors, reflecting back a myriad of distorted images. Confused about the reasons for original placements and emotionally bruised from further moves between foster homes, youth in care have many unresolved questions about their identity (McFadden, 1984a).

Geiser reports:

A teenage boy who was placed when he was two drew up a list of questions that he wanted answered about his past that illustrates this loss of self as a person.

1. What hospital was I born in? What was my birth weight? At what time of day was I born?
2. Are there any old pictures of me when I was small?
3. What did my parents do for a living? Are there any pictures of them in my record?
4. Do I have brothers and sisters? Any close relatives, like aunts or uncles?
5. Do I have any godparents? Who witnessed my baptism?
6. Do I have a middle name?
7. What were the names of some of my foster parents in the homes I lived in? My doctors? My teachers? My social workers?

8. Was I sick a lot as a child? What sicknesses did I have? Did I have any accidents or broken bones?
9. Why did I have to leave all the places I was in and why am I here?
10. Do I belong to anybody? (Geiser, 1973, p. 69)

Many youth have lost their historical roots; the present is cluttered with distorted images resulting in a confused sense of time, place and self. Some youth in care may be confused about things as fundamental as their own family names. Fanshel and Shinn (1978) reported that 26 percent of children studied could not give their mothers' names, and 22 percent could not give their fathers' names. Festinger (1983) describes the confusion of youngsters wondering whether to go by their foster families' names. Although 61.9 percent chose not to use any name but their own, 21 percent had wanted to use a foster family's name, and 17 percent spoke of calling themselves by their foster families' names. They expressed great concern about needing more background information on their families with 50 percent describing themselves as having no roots. Children in transcultural placements noted particular confusion (Festinger, 1983).

In several studies children in foster care or youth formerly in care voiced concerns about being different or set apart as a result of their foster status. Festinger (1983) describes close to 63 percent of her respondents as feeling different. Experiences which served as reminders of being different included using the clinic (rather than the foster family's regular doctor), agency rules and procedures, and caseworker visits to school. Some respondents also cited feelings of being treated like an outsider by foster parents or the biological children of foster parents, who "never let me forget I was in foster care . . . that I was not as good as they" (p. 265). Fanshel and Shinn (1978) noted that almost 25 percent of their subjects perceived differential treatment. In thinking about how foster care is different from one's own family, the subjects mentioned issues such as clothes, money, fights, and not being able to go places where other children could go. In the Jones and Moses (1984) study, 43 percent of subjects reported feeling they had been treated differently by the foster parents, other children, school teachers, relatives, and people in the community.

Poor self-esteem is reflected in, and compounded by, foster children's school problems. Many studies report that youth in foster care lag educationally or have difficulties in school learning and school adjustment (Jones and Moses, 1984; Gil and Bogart, 1982; Shapiro, 1970; Festinger, 1983; Gruber, 1978; Rice and Semmelroth, 1968). School is to children and youth as work is to adults. Most young people in care would like to do well in school and be accepted in the culture of their peers. Chaotic histories of school changes and varying educational expectations of the different foster families leave the child confused and wary. Worries about school and subsequent poor performance lead foster children to limited career and work aspirations.

Another issue which reappears thematically is fear of punishment, maltreatment, or abuse. At a foster care retreat a girl confided, "I told my worker and my legal aid attorney that the man who was then my foster father was sexually abusing me. They promised to do something. That was months ago and I'm not in that home no more but he is still a foster parent" (Barnett, 1985, p. 5). A study done by Jones and Moses (1984) indicated that 21 percent of subjects were whipped or punished in a severe way by foster parents, and 9 percent had someone in the foster home try to take advantage of them sexually. Studies of substantiated maltreatment in family foster care indicate rates between two incidents per thousand and 26 per thousand foster homes (Ryan, 1983; Vera Institute of Justice, 1981). Youth in foster care may have worried a great deal about actual or potential maltreatment, but they rarely confide in the worker, and often do not speak of the maltreatment until they have reached adulthood and moved out of the foster care system (McFadden, 1984b). This in part may be explained by their negative perceptions of themselves. Since they view themselves as bad and unworthy, they may expect maltreatment.

The Independent Living Project at Eastern Michigan University is an attempt to focus equally on tangible and intangible skills. The emotional and moral developmental needs of youth emancipation are stressed along with self-help and employment skills. The project provides a curriculum to train foster parents as primary teachers in the preparation of youth for independent living, a second curriculum for the youth to develop skills under the tutelage of their foster parents, and a structured sequence of group activities for emancipating youth. Leaving home again is a major theme throughout the curriculum and a central focus of one module. This helps foster parents and youth comprehend and face the complex issues of loss and loss of identity which underlie adjustment to emancipation.

THEMES OF THE EMANCIPATION PROCESS

In working with youth facing emancipation one must be equally aware both of the obvious real concerns youth face and the subtle undercurrents which may be operating just outside of their consciousness. As foster parents become aware of these subterranean influences on youth in care, a great deal of formerly inexplicable behavior begins to make sense. Foster parents find greater empathy and compassion.

A major theme is the likelihood that preparation for emancipation will lead to *reactivation of earlier losses*. Usually a youth is not aware of the connection between present behavior and earlier losses. The extent to which a given youth should be helped to develop this awareness is a clinical question to be handled by the youth's therapist. However, foster parents can come to understand the importance of their supportive role and the need to work closely with the therapist, rather than doing the uncovering themselves.

A girl who had been placed at an early age due to the death of her mother had apparently blamed herself for her mother's death. When she began preparing for independent living in a foster home where she felt relatively secure after a series of short lived placements, she became beset with anxiety about her foster mother's health. When she moved from the foster home, she became profoundly sad and telephoned the foster mother frequently. One night, when the girl was in crisis, she hugged her foster mother and sobbed, "I'm afraid you'll die if I'm not there to take care of you." The foster mother shared this with the therapist and caseworker, and they were able to piece together the unconscious trauma which the girl was re-living.

It is equally important for foster parents—and other members of the team—to understand the theme of *maladaptive responses to separation and rejection*. Most youth leaving foster care have had more than one placement. Typically there was at least one placement which had not worked out, perhaps several. Many youth report confusion about leaving foster homes. One youth stated, "I never could figure it out. I came home from school one day feeling pretty good and there was the worker. My bag was packed and my foster mom didn't even hang around to say good-bye. The worker didn't explain to me what I had done wrong or why I had to move." Many youth act out the self-loathing and self-blame they feel from the big trauma, the departure from their family of origin. Each move becomes a reenactment of the original pain. Some learn to send up a barrage of self-protecting distancing behavior whenever they feel threatened that a foster parent is becoming too involved with them. Others run away. Still others provoke abuse and rejection (Littner, 1960; McFadden, 1984b).

Foster parents need help understanding that when a youth is preparing to leave the foster home, the process can trigger a reenactment of past departures or an acting out of an overt or repressed identification with a biological parent. Some youth set themselves up and provoke the foster parent into asking them to leave early. Others choose a maladaptive behavior, such as becoming pregnant or engaging in criminal activity, as a way of asserting kinship with a parent who did the same thing. Occasionally, foster parents may assist the youth through a variation of "Please don't eat the daisies" by identifying for troubled youngsters the behavior that will lead to their rejection:

> A foster parent of a seventeen-year-old girl told her, "I'm pretty tolerant and I plan to stick with you until you are ready to be on your own. There's only one thing I won't stand for. That is bringing dope into my home." The foster parent supported the girl through several crises until the young woman was working and preparing to leave. When she left a bag of

marijuana obviously placed on the dining table, the foster mother felt compelled to have her leave immediately. Thus the girl brought about the rejection she had felt years earlier from her own family.

Foster parents and the treatment team also need to be sensitized to the potency of *reunion fantasies* as the emancipation process winds toward its inevitable conclusion. Many youth in care cherish a secret belief that their parents really loved them and wanted them, but that the intervention of the evil caseworker or judge prevented the parent from reclaiming the child. This resolute denial wards off the self-blame engendered by the separation. Other youth may more realistically acknowledge the shortcomings of their parents but hope for a dramatic change in the relationship. The farther down the emancipation road the youth goes, the more vulnerable he or she becomes as the agency and foster home are relinquished as a source of security. One often finds that the intensity of the reunion fantasy seems to be proportional to the degree of insecurity the youth is feeling at the moment.

Part of the developmental task of the older youth/younger adult is formation of identity (Erikson, 1959), or differentiation from the family of origin (Laird, 1978). How is a youth to either claim or repudiate aspects of a parent if there has been no opportunity to engage in contact with the parent? It seems almost inevitable that most youth in foster care harbor reunion fantasies and that many will act on them. It is very important for the agency and foster parents to help a youth develop a more realistic understanding of the circumstances which brought him or her into care, and to facilitate contact with the family when appropriate:

Amelia, age 18, believed that her mother would welcome her home with open arms, and confided to her foster mother her secret plan to arrive, unannounced, at her mother's home and tell her that she had come home to stay. The worker and therapist were aware of the mother's extreme rejection and wanted Amelia to realize the reality of her situation while she was still in the relative security of her foster home. They arranged a meeting with the mother. After Amelia made several overtures for affection, her mother said, "I didn't want you then, and I don't want you now. Please get out of my life and go your own way." Amelia responded to this rejection with near suicidal depression, but she said to her foster parent, "I'm glad this happened now while I was with you and had a therapist to talk to. If I'd been out on my own, and went to my mother for help, I probably would have killed myself."

A final theme of leaving home again is enhancing ability to accept the past and develop *emotional scar tissue*. They are poised anxiously on the brink, ready for a leap into adulthood. All muscles are tensed, all energy is focused on what lies ahead. They do not want to open old wounds or bring up sadness from the past. They are far too insecure to let down their defenses for the type of uncovering associated with intensive therapy. While the treatment team may recognize many residuals from the past in present behavior, the team needs to help youth maintain a focus on the here and now, and their goals for the near future:

One young woman verbalized in group,

> It's kind of like learning to ride a bicycle. When you're getting ready to go on your own, you need to get everything coordinated and to keep your balance even if you wobble a little. If you look back at where you've been you may fall off. You need to look at where you're going. Of course, it might not hurt, once you really got rolling, to peek in your rearview mirror to see if anything is sneaking up on you.

TREATMENT TEAM ROLES
IN PREPARING YOUTH FOR EMANCIPATION

The treatment team consists minimally of the foster parent and social worker. Under optimal circumstances the team also includes a therapist and a youth group leader. Each member plays a role in the preparation process. Each helps the emancipating youth handle the complex tasks of leaving home again. Coordination of the team is critical. Each member helps, in a slightly different way, as the youth struggles with his or her adaptation to increasing independence.

Worker Tasks

The worker has a number of important tasks, not the least of which is the identification of youth in need of preparation for independent living at an early enough age that adequate time is allowed for skill building and relationship building. If the youth is not in counseling, a referral should be made at the time the youth enters the phase of active preparation for emancipation.

If the agency asks the foster parent to begin training the youth in life skills and enrolls him or her in a support group, whether it is two years or six months before the emancipation date, this will raise the issue of leaving home again. Reactive depression may begin at the time the youth begins anticipating leaving rather than when she or he actually leaves. The worker should be prepared to deal with these symptoms and help the youth resolve their feelings.

If the young person has been in multiple placements, it is the worker's responsibility to develop a complete placement record, with names, addresses and dates, so that the youth can clear up any confusion about where he or she was at any given age. As much as possible, the worker should assemble a few key facts regarding each placement family so the youth will be able to organize various memories. Letters from former foster parents detailing anecdotes about the youth and photographs are useful additions. They enable the youth to reconstruct her or his identity during the turbulent years.

During the years prior to emancipation, the worker should continue to review permanence planning to determine if return to the family or adoption might yet be possible. If reunification with parents is impossible, the worker should seek other ways to strengthen ties with the family of origin. Intensive work around the youth's relationship with the family should be done in order to help the youth deal with reunion fantasies and avoid the heartbreak of later rejection. If young people must relinquish this fantasy once and for all, it is better to do it at a time when they still have access to agency services. This clears the air for more realistic planning for independent living.

Each youth should have an opportunity to sit down with a worker and discuss why he or she is still in care and why independence rather than return home is the plan. Worker, youth, and foster parents should plan together how the youth will live after leaving care. They should discuss employment opportunities, use of entitlement programs, location of housing and any other services needed. The plan should be realistically based on the competence and desires of the youth and the availability of resources. Many young people will require sustained worker advocacy to locate scholarship funds or to determine eligibility for various programs. Some will need ongoing adult mental health services. To meet these needs, a worker may have to learn new systems with all the convoluted issues of eligibility, entitlement, and communication across systems boundaries.

The worker must also identify the youth's need for treatment and receptivity to treatment. Young people who have been in the system for many years have often been through many different types of therapy and may have had more treatment than needed. They have learned the treatment lingo. Others react violently, fearful of being labeled crazy. It is useful if treatment is explained as a way the youth can gain support as she or he goes through the process of moving toward independence.

Therapist's Role

The therapist will be kept busy helping the youth deal with his or her anger and sorrow and facilitating the mourning process triggered by the losses surfacing as a result of contemplating leaving home again. Most youth approaching emancipation are able to at least glimpse the concept that

> physical separations or death need not be experienced as permanently irretrievable losses. One's memories of those lost others can keep them very much alive and they, therefore, remain a significant part of one, which indeed they are . . . a moving and profoundly integrative experience. (Colon, 1973, p. 434)

Tooley (1978) speaks of the importance of an inner treasury

> resembling the hodge-podge that every latency-age child
> stores in a carton under the bed: souvenirs and bottle caps and
> trophies and photographs and . . . things that have symbolic
> value in their own right, things that have the capacity for stim-
> ulating pleasant memories, and things that reinforce a trea-
> sured mythology of the self. (p. 175)

Work with a life story book, or its equivalent, can help the youth
sort through the jumble of a fragmented past and pull together a
warmer sense of self. By helping the young person sift through the
past or look in the rearview mirror (while riding the bicycle full
speed ahead), the therapist supports the youth's efforts in the here
and now.

Group Work

Support groups for youth are an important tool for implementing
the independent living curriculum and providing an opportunity to
enhance social skills in preparation for *inter*dependence. No one
living independently really makes it on one's own (Maluccio,
1985). Each youth needs a repertoire of social skills to develop a
supportive social network. A group is an excellent medium through
which to learn that one is not so different as one supposes. Activities which involve making choices and defining the self increase a
youth's sense of autonomy. Creative activity using clay, paint, paper, and other media allow for expression of pent-up feelings. Team
or small group activities such as building a tower with blocks or
planning a social event are equally useful to youth in fostering the
sort of cooperation they will need for the future. The activities of
the group augment both the therapy and the training provided by the
youth curriculum.

Foster Parent Role

Foster parents are in a critical position to teach the tangible skills
needed for leaving home. Foster parents provide the practical
know-how for teaching about first aid and menu planning. They
also have a role in helping with the intangible skills. When address-

ing the complex issues facing a youth leaving home again, much of the foster parents' role focuses on providing empathetic support and understanding. Some of the foster parent tasks module include being interviewed by the youth on how it felt for the foster parent to leave home; helping youth assemble memorabilia and talismans whether in a life story book or in a tote bag; and working to determine what their ongoing relationship will be after the youth departs. The foster parent must also assess the impact of their own ambivalence and the youth's ambivalence about leaving. Just as foster parents must understand the stress inherent in a youth's entry into the foster home (Wilkes, 1974), they also need to understand and manage the impact of a youth's departure on the entire family. In order to manage this transition and to empower the youth to handle the separation appropriately, foster parents are encouraged to assist the youth in determining just how he or she wants to spend the last day in the foster home. The plan might include a favorite dish to be served at dinner, a special activity for all to enjoy together, or the way the youth wishes to handle saying good-bye. Foster parents are encouraged to consider the importance of ritual in marking transitions and to develop a ritual which fits their family. It might involve baking a cake or lighting a candle, singing a song or potting a plant. Emphasis is not on the type of ritual, but rather on the *process* of developing that which is unique and suits the needs of the youth and the foster family. It must be specific for one given family in the same way as certain rules are specific for each family (Palazolli et al., 1977). By placing the youth in charge of managing the leaving-home-again event, the foster parent helps the youth undo old patterns of separation/rejection and resolve some of the pain of earlier losses while supporting feelings of autonomy.

RESPONSIBILITY TO YOUTH POST-EMANCIPATION

Although some youth return to seek support from foster parents or caseworkers at various times during their young adulthood, there are few programs or formal services available during this critical period of development. Caseworkers and foster parents know that one's parental responsibility to their own children does not end when a youth turns eighteen or finishes high school. Throughout early adulthood, young people return to their parents' home in times of crisis, for vacations, or to plan weddings. Young adults typically ask for assistance with planning major purchases such as an automobile or a home. They want grandparental support in babysitting and nurturing their children. Former foster children do not have the advantage of a secure base from which to emancipate. They need to define what is the home they will turn to for support and clarify the extent to which their foster parents are willing to assume an ongoing quasi-parental role. All too often former foster children are out on the proverbial limb, cut off from their families of origin, but no longer part of the foster family. At a time when powerful identity issues surface, the youth may need to return to a trusted counselor or therapist. At a point in the life cycle when the youth is purposefully or accidentally faced with impending parenthood, again many unresolved issues from the past surface. Before a young woman can mother she must come to terms with what her mother did to her, and how she will be different.

The agonies and triumphs of the young adult years are a compelling rationale for the provision of follow-up services for young adults who have left the system. Such long-term services would acknowledge and help compensate for the difficulties of leaving home *again*.

Chapter 11

Therapeutic Foster Parent: Professionally or Emotionally Involved Parent?

Juanita N. Baker

ABSTRACT. Training can help foster parents manage reactions to the foster child, avoid stress and burnout, and cope with the difficult times so that placement is sustained. Training is necessary so foster parents will not take the child's aggressive behavior personally, will avoid becoming embroiled in power struggles, and will be less likely to become hurt or embarrassed by the child's behavior. Training will involve individual consultation by the social worker as well as participation in a foster parent group. Staff will assist foster parents to develop behavioral management and communication skills as well as their own coping and self-control skills. Foster parents are given permission to take care of their own needs, are assisted in developing stress management skills, learn how to increase their own self-esteem, and learn to use cognitive approaches to handle their own emotions. Foster parents develop an understanding that they cannot change the child's behavior but can only change the way which they respond to the child, which may provide the child opportunities to change his or her own behavior.

Juanita N. Baker is Assistant Professor of Psychology, and Coordinator, Therapeutic Foster Home Program, School of Psychology, Florida Institute of Technology, 150 West University Boulevard, Melbourne, FL 32901.

The Florida Institute of Technology's (FIT) Therapeutic Foster Home Program (TFHP) is partially funded by the State of Florida Department of Health and Rehabilitative Services. Grateful acknowledgement is made to Michael Healy for his editorial suggestions and TFHP parents and FIT staff for sharing their thoughts on ways to help TFHP parents cope with their job.

One of the difficulties of therapeutic foster care (TFC) programs is keeping children in placement. Most foster parents think of giving up the emotionally disturbed child within the first 90 days of placement or after a relapse when the child's behavior gets out of control. How do some parents manage to get through these trying periods maintaining their sense of perspective, humor, and commitment, whereas others become overly emotionally involved? Vulnerable parents take the child's aggressive behavior personally, become excessively embroiled in power struggles, become hurt or embarrassed by the youth's behavior and become increasingly stressed with each crisis. At first it is always difficult for the parents. It takes time for parents to effect change in the lives of their foster children. Dramatic improvement is possible yet not without much effort and stress. In time the parent can recognize the progress and feel a sense of accomplishment as well as feel that living with the child is tolerable. This paper will address what trainers can do to reinforce and inspire the parent until that day arrives.

Most TFC programs are primarily concerned with the treatment of children. However, to insure that work with parents is maximally successful, TFC professionals must place more emphasis upon dealing with the special needs of the parents themselves. Probably the most important factor in keeping the child in placement is to teach the parents the most viable and effective parenting/therapeutic techniques to effect rapid behavioral change. We teach both behavior modification skills (Becker, 1971; Clark, 1985; Fleischman, Horne & Arthur, 1983) and communication skills (Gordon, 1970; Bolton, 1979). It is important to help them immediately see that change is possible. After applying the new skills, one trainee remarked, "These effective skills are a primary antidote for burnout." Learning therapeutic skills helps them control their own behavior toward the child. They learn to "act, not just react."

We attempt to communicate to the TFC parents that they should not only be loving parents but also professional therapeutic change agents. After parents are trained in therapeutic and teaching techniques, they become active members of our treatment team and exert control in decisions in which they are involved. When the child is placed in their home (with their approval), they are involved in behavioral analysis, monitoring behaviors, treatment planning and implementing methods and skills learned in the training sessions. The specification of very definite goals and recording the child's behavior (whether the target behavior occurred that day or not) as well as their own (whether they used the planned intervention technique or not that day) helps the parents see their role as professional, more effectively track and modify problem behaviors, and keep a record revealing the step-by-step progress of the child. One parent remarked, "When I tracked behaviors it made me think more of what I was doing and how I might respond differently." Requiring the parent to briefly measure how they are doing at maintaining the professional role or feeling in control versus becoming emotionally involved and burning out provides feedback to the staff. If the crisis can be seen to be building in the earlier phases, the staff can more readily provide timely parent support, arrange for respite or other needs to be met, and provide more intensive counseling or family therapy for troubled areas or unresolved issues. Their professional role also entails keeping treatment records, attending weekly consultation sessions with their supervisor, and coordinating the treatment plan with their case manager, physician, and school or community agency personnel. Addressing them as professional parents from the beginning helps them identify with their new role.

Monthly therapeutic foster parent meetings are held to encourage consultation and peer support. Recognizing that other parents are also dealing with extreme behaviors has been valuable to our TFC parents. We try to provide an open atmosphere. We stress that it is OK to make mistakes and not know all the answers. Mistakes can be corrected. The child won't experience irreparable harm if we are warm, open, and honest. We recognize and want the parents to also see that they are doing the best they can with the knowledge, skills, and understanding they have at the time. They deserve much credit.

A strong emotional bond between our staff persons and the TFC parents develops through at least weekly contact and the building of mutual respect. The availability of 24-hour consultation and provision of these support services helps TFC parents maintain the line between professional and distraught parent. One of our staff remarked, "I'm spending more time doing therapy with the professional parent than the biological parent!" In all families persons have vulnerable spots (of course, there are no perfect parents), which may have to be dealt with during placement before they can handle certain aspects of these difficult children. In times of crisis it is important to provide that needed support. It is much easier to do this if concepts necessary for their own control or stress reduction have been taught previously during the training.

The staff must give the parent therapeutic skills but they also must teaching coping and self-control skills and address parental concerns, attitudes, and needs. Having TFC parents keep a loose-leaf notebook which contains the handouts from our training and continuing education as well as their own personal growth home-work exercises helps the parent recapture their more recently learned perspective when in crisis. As an example, the handout "Strategies to Prevent Burnout" is included at the end of this chapter and summarizes for the parent the variety of approaches they may use in handling their own problems and maintaining a professional attitude and role.

We have found Fleischman, Horne, and Arthur's (1983) problem-solving steps ("What is my goal? What am I doing now? Is what I'm doing helping me to achieve my goal? If it isn't, what do I need to do differently?") have helped our parents focus on the task at hand, decide what is most therapeutic to do at any particular time, and more calmly implement intervention skills.

The professional therapeutic parents are taught and given permission to take care of their own needs. They are urged to maintain feelings of self-worth. Using Maslow's (1954) hierarchy of needs, parents make a list of how they satisfy each of their own needs. This helps them understand that the child has the same needs and it is valuable for everyone to ask directly for what they want. This openness and honesty will reduce the deviousness and manipulation frequently exhibited by fearful children. We emphasize the importance of making sure that their own, their spouse's and their own children's needs are satisfied so that they will have energy to love and give to the foster child. This helps reduce guilt to arrange time for these needs.

Stress management skills—setting priorities, time scheduling, and relaxation techniques (Fleischman et al., 1983) are taught. It is expected that the child will be their primary unpredictable stressor. Arranging for respite, weekly child care, and vacations is essential.

Some of our parents who have decided not to take a child full-time have been helpful in providing respite. We encourage putting fun, privacy, and relaxation into their lives. Showing them that there is a logic to the stages in placement (i.e., honeymoon period, testing the limits phase, working on one problem at a time until each is handled adequately, transition, termination) helps a parent look forward to passing through the stage, rather than thinking that it is a permanent stressful situation.

We review the reasons and motivations for their being a foster parent and recognize (and give permission) for some of their needs to be met through their professional parenting. Although there should be rewards and satisfactions for being a TFC parent, we urge them not to depend on the child to satisfy these needs totally. They list their social and emotional support, i.e., those whom they are loved by and love as well as those persons they can call upon who will aid them when in need (including calling upon the primary staff consultant or our program back-up person, available on a 24-hour basis).

To strengthen their own self-esteem, TFC parents learn cognitive techniques to identify negative self-talk and learn talking back to themselves in positive ways. They make a list of their own strengths, the professional techniques used well, their accomplishments and review these lists periodically. We have found that having these written down in their notebooks enhances self-esteem especially after difficult stressful periods. One of our basic therapeutic principles is to "leave the child feeling good about themselves in every situation." Training focuses on ways to build self-esteem (Reasoner, 1982) for the professional parent as well as for the child. Reasoner argues that building self-esteem includes providing a sense of trust by being honest in all ways, a sense of identity by recognizing one's uniqueness and strengths, a sense of belonging by working and playing together, a sense of purpose by setting goals, and a sense of personal competence by taking responsibility, making decisions, and being reinforced for a job well done. Parents and children are encouraged to accept their past actions and to be responsible for them but foremost to leave the past behind and focus on what actions they now can take to make themselves feel good.

A cognitive approach to handling their own emotions is presented to the parents. The basic emotions (hurt, anger, fear, love, guilt, depression, and happiness) which the parents will be handling as well as experiencing can be seen as falling under one of several categories varying in intensity. For example, under the category anger, the emotions could range from irritation, frustration, resentment, hatred, to fury, but the basic thought underlying each of them is that "that person shouldn't have done that to me." When TFC parents identify their thoughts, they can identify their emotions; or if they are feeling deeply, they can search for the relevant thoughts causing their distress. This simplification helps make emotions more understandable and they discover they have a choice of what they think. As a result, parents can exercise greater control over their emotions. Of course, if they can see this thought/feeling sequence for themselves, they are more likely to be able to understand the child's feelings and thoughts too, reflecting and helping the child to understand themselves.

Ellis (1962), Beck (1976), Meichenbaum (1977), and Kanfer (1975) have emphasized the importance of our cognitions on influencing affect and behavior. All parents become emotionally involved with the child in their home, but it is possible to help parents not take the child's behavior personally and to not own the child's problem. Parents are taught cognitive techniques for handling crises especially when they are being blamed and rejected by the child. Alternative ways of viewing the youth's problem and attitudes which facilitate handling the child with philosophical detachment are discussed. TFC parents are asked the following questions: What positive thoughts would help you take a professional role? What have you gained from being a TFC parent? What kind of thinking would facilitate your staying emotionally detached so you can be an effective therapeutic change agent? To maximize insight, it is helpful to arrange to have parents as a group discuss their answers to these questions. As parents become experienced, they can look back and share with the new parents the attitudes that were previously not helpful.

A list of negative thoughts with which previous TF parents have had difficulties is presented. These thoughts illustrate taking an emotionally involved, perfectionistic, and rigid attitude towards the child and crises. With the goal of helping the parents change their attitudes, we ask them these questions as each negative thought is reviewed: What behaviors of your child could automatically stimulate this thought? Now why might believing this idea cause you problems in handling the child? Why might these be problematic thoughts which would interfere with your professional role? Just identifying these thoughts and the fact that they may negatively impact on the child has helped our parents look at their own cognitive patterns more carefully. This introspection has helped them avoid blaming the child. Parents are encouraged to analyze their thinking patterns and to try thinking up their own counterarguments.

A primary error many TFC parents (as well as therapists) make is that they think they can control and change the child's behavior. Although the goal is to change the child's behavior, TFC parents may be misled into thinking that they are responsible for changing the child's behavior, when they are actually responsible for only changing their own behavior which may then influence the choices that the child makes. Grasping this concept helps TFC parents relax more and focus on how they might set up the antecedent and consequent conditions to facilitate the child's positive growth choices.

Parents thrive on reinforcement and recognition which can be given at every opportunity: verbally in telephone contacts, weekly supervision, monthly newsletter, at monthly meetings, occasional letters specifically for the purpose of praising them, and in communications to the funding agency. Our staff points out the parents' strengths, their professional and therapeutic actions, and contributions to colleagues and family and their efforts to set up the growth conditions for the particular child. This encourages parents to renew and maintain their commitment.

SUMMARY

The TFC program staff can do much to train, prepare, and encourage parents to take a professional role and maintain detachment from the child. Our program encourages parents to utilize therapeutic skills, monitor the child's and their own behaviors, develop behavioral treatment plans and emphasizes that the parents should take care of their own needs. We also try to teach TFC parents to handle their emotions and employ cognitive techniques to examine their professional and emotional attitudes towards the child. Parents report that our approach helps them better manage the inevitable crises and withstand the tendency to give up, and just as importantly, be a more effective therapeutic change agent to meet the primary goal of helping youth live up to their potential.

APPENDIX

STRATEGIES TO PREVENT BURNOUT   Juanita N. Baker, Ph.D. @1985

---

1.   TAKE CARE OF YOUR OWN NEEDS (Check Maslow's hierarchy. How are you doing? Health, sleep, nutrition, exercise, safety, love, self-esteem, use   potential, creativity)

2.   REDUCE STRESS by not overscheduling yourself or family (Can you arrange things in the   environment to make it easier?). Set aside times for relaxation, privacy.

3.   Love, belonging needs, form CLOSE, INTIMATE RELATIONSHIPS, arrange for peer support:(have at least 4)   a. spouse, children, relatives, neighbors
              b. close friends (talk about something other than foster care)
              c. other foster parents, join TFHP monthly meetings. and Brevard County
                 Foster Parents Association, your supervisor
              d. religious and/or extracurricular activities groups

4.   COMPETENCY: review skills, handouts, to refine skills, gain new ideas, skills: Decide what changes need to be made. Continue learning, growing, developing your talents.

5.   TAKE TIME FOR FUN, plan variety and excitement into your life. Get involved! Take a moment to smell the roses, view the sunset, appreciate the child, listen to the music, feel the sunshine, and taste the meal...use every sense.
Spread a little of your sunshine every day!

6.   Take RESPITE: arrange for child care sitters for an evening or afternoon off weekly, an occasional weekend, and a yearly vacation.

7.   Use relaxation techniques and/or get physical EXERCISE.

8.   Use PROBLEM SOLVING steps daily and for crises:
              Step One: What is my goal?
              Step Two: What am I doing now?
              Step Three: Is what I'm doing helping me to achieve my goal?
              Step Four: If it isn't, what do I need to do differently?

9.   ATTITUDE: detached (keep the child's problems separate from your self-esteem), caring for the child's pain (the child is doing the best job he/she knows how to satisfy his/her own needs) a desire to use skills to help

10.   Obtain our professional help and support--regularly CONSULT US on a weekly basis, not just in time of crisis. TELL US , WE'RE A TEAM.

APPENDIX (continued)

11.   Review your list of reasons, motivation for entering foster care; your VALUES and PRIORITIES.

12.   Focus on YOUR STRENGTHS, the child's and your family's positives; your "highs"

13.   Remember YOUR ACCOMPLISHMENTS personally and with the child
      a. review the child's treatment plan
      b. look at the data. What changes have you made?
      c. remember that small steps will lead to big steps
          (the child took a long time to become what he/she is:
          San Francisco wasn't rebuilt in a day, but it was started!)

Chapter 12

Doing It in Public:
A Review of Foster Family
Treatment Program Development
in Missouri

Brad Bryant
Fred Simmens
Mary McKee

ABSTRACT. Foster family treatment programs have been developed primarily by private agencies, although public efforts have helped shape the model. Public programs, however, increasingly are becoming involved in the development of programs of this kind. The Missouri Division of Family Services is one of the few public agencies to sponsor a statewide pilot program of foster family treatment. The Division's experience offers valuable lessons and practical guidance regarding the development of treatment foster care in the public sector.

Developing a new program within an existing organization is a difficult task. To begin a new program within a public agency where external scrutiny and internal political pressures strongly impact daily decision making and job performance is an even greater challenge; one which can be further complicated by sheer organiza-

Brad Bryant is Director of Research and Training at People Places, Inc., 1215 N. Augusta Street, Staunton, VA 24401. Fred Simmens is Supervisor, Program Specialist Unit, Missouri Division of Family Services, Post Office Box 68, Jefferson City, MO 65103. Mary McKee is Special Service Supervisor III, Missouri Division of Family Services, 615 East 17th Street, Kansas City, MO 64106.

tion size and the consequent inertial symptoms of bureaucratic bulge. Public agencies are, despite the difficulty of the task, developing new programs in the area of treatment foster family care which has been dominated by private sector service providers. Some of these recent public initiatives seem to be meeting with success and promise both to survive and grow. This paper will share the experience and learning from a two-year effort in developing a statewide pilot program of foster family treatment (FFT) in Missouri.

WHY DO IT IN PUBLIC?

Organizations are dynamic human systems. Whenever a new element is introduced the entire system is affected. Adjustments must be made where the new part interfaces with other units, departments, or individuals. Various policies and practices must be altered to make room psychologically and technically for new procedures and personnel. Authority, status, and power relationships may be disturbed. A new equilibrium must be achieved. In short, change must occur; and change is unsettling.

The challenge of developing a new program within a large public bureaucracy goes well beyond the specific tasks of designing and implementing the program itself. New program development is an exercise in organization change in which the impact on the larger system must be carefully considered and addressed as a fundamental element of the development plan. Change efforts are facilitated by such organizational characteristics as flexibility, responsiveness, open communications and an organization culture which values creativity and entrepreneurship (Deal & Kennedy, 1982). Large bureaucratic organizations do not typically present these characteristics. Size itself creates a degree of inertia, resistance to change, and a by-the-book rigidity antithetical to innovation. Bureaucracies tend to be strongly hierarchical, protective of the status quo, and famous for red tape bottlenecks which leave change efforts locked in standing committees or full file cabinets.

Change efforts in public versus private bureaucracies are even harder to effect. Public agencies generally are subject to closer public scrutiny and stronger political pressure than private organizations dedicated to the same tasks. The fish-bowled environment of many public service agencies breeds caution, conservatism, and conformity—none of which are conducive to the development of innovative new programs (Sayles, 1979).

Given the obstacles to developing new service programs in public bureaucracies, one might question whether such programs as foster family treatment should be attempted at all by the public sector. Private providers have pioneered the development of what is an emerging foster family treatment model (Bryant, 1980). Private programs generally are smaller, more open in communication, more flexible and entrepreneurial than public agencies. They are more likely to have staff with skills and experience in the treatment technologies needed for foster family treatment than public agencies. Many states have chosen already to contract for foster family treatment services rather than attempt to create such services themselves. There are sound precedents for full or partial privatization of some public services in this country and solid reasons for continuing and expanding such arrangements (Nigro & Nigro, 1977; Amara, 1979; Charpie, 1979; Toffler, 1980; Bryant, 1983). There are several compelling reasons, however, for public agencies to become more closely involved in the provision of foster family treatment services either directly or in partnership with the private sector.

First is the reality of responsibility for providing care and treatment to disturbed youth needing out-of-home placements. While public agencies may refer their wards to private foster family treatment programs, those programs are not obliged to accept them. A private program may not have an appropriate treatment foster family with whom to place the child despite the fact that the child may be appropriate for foster family treatment. Given choice and adequate referrals, private programs may choose to work with the less difficult youngsters referred to them, leaving the public custodial agencies with the responsibility to provide placement and treatment for the most disturbed youth in their communities. Without a foster family treatment program of its own, the custodial agency is faced with two familiar choices. They may continue to place more disturbed youth inappropriately in regular foster care which typically does not provide stability or continuity of care for such children

(Pardeck, 1982), or they may place these youngsters in costly residential treatment centers which often are more restrictive and less normalizing than needed.

A second practical reason for public agencies to consider direct provision of foster family treatment is the simple absence of such services where they are clearly needed. Missouri's program was developed because of the lack of public or private community-based treatment programs in the state and the growing pressure by localities for residential placements of children who could not be managed in regular foster care. The public sector took the lead in foster family treatment largely because the private sector could not.

A final reason favoring public sector involvement in foster family treatment relates to the foster family care system as a whole and to the changing needs of the children it currently serves. In the ten years since passage of Public Law 96-272, the number of children placed in foster homes has decreased dramatically in many states. This is due primarily to the increased emphasis on preventing out-of-home placements and keeping birth families together. An unanticipated result of the progress in this area in some states is that those children who now enter foster care are older, have had longer exposure to pathological family situations, and present more severe problems than children in care a decade ago. The state of Virginia offers an example. Between 1975 and 1985, the number of children in foster family care was reduced by nearly half (Virginia Department of Social Services, 1986). The difference between the two foster care populations, however, goes beyond total number in care. In 1975, 37 percent of children in the foster family system had entered care at age 13 or older. In 1985, 72 percent of the children in care were teenagers at time of entry. Foster children entering care in 1985 presented significantly higher frequencies of single and multiple emotional/behavioral problems, parent-child conflicts, substance abuse and delinquency compared to a 1975 foster care population sample (Virginia Department of Social Services, 1986). Similar findings are indicated for children in Washington, D.C. and elsewhere around the nation (Jordan, 1986).

Studies of foster family placement and continuity of care show that older children with moderate to severe emotional or behavioral problems adjust least well to regular foster family care (Pardeck,

1982; Fanshel & Shinn, 1978). Increasingly, however, these are the children we see entering foster family care. While the numbers are fewer, the needs of current foster children appear to be greater than children in care in decades past. These children require not only a caring home environment, but systematic treatment and social skills training in and out of the foster home. Their foster parents need on-going training, support and technical assistance, crisis intervention services and higher pay to attract and retain them in undertaking a more professionalized, change agent role with children. Line workers need lower caseloads and greater technical expertise in behavior analysis, in-home treatment program planning, social skills training and other therapeutic skills. The service elements needed for dealing with severely troubled youth in foster family care generally are the same elements which define the foster family treatment model.

The organization and delivery of traditional foster family care must change given the changing nature and needs of today's foster care population. That change will need to be in the direction of foster family treatment. Public agencies can help create alternative community-based services for the more difficult youth they serve by developing programs of foster family treatment and also can lay the foundation for the more intensive type of foster family care that will be required to meet the needs of all children in foster home placements.

TECHNICAL ASSISTANCE
FOR PROGRAM DEVELOPMENT

People Places, Inc., a private, nonprofit foster family treatment program begun in 1973, has been active in assisting new foster family treatment program development since the late 1970s. Considerable research, resource development and support-building must be completed, however, before any outside technical assistance is given or before implementation of any specific service model is begun. Program developers often are buffeted on the one hand by pressures from above or outside the agency for early implementation and on the other by legitimate or inertial pressures from within the agency to slow down.

A sound replication model alone, even if accompanied by substantial and effective expert assistance, will not guarantee a successful foster family treatment program. The organizational hierarchy must be worked to gain top-level support and commitment of adequate resources. This will require thorough research into the rationale and data supporting foster family treatment generally, into specific program models and the resources needed to mount effective programs. Collateral support within the sponsoring agency will be needed from staff whose work is affected by the new program or whose authority or status may be impacted by it. Understanding of and commitment to the foster family treatment model must be developed by staff within the sponsoring agency before the program can be sold to others whose support and cooperation are essential (e.g., treatment foster parents, other community service agencies). These efforts are likely to require much more time than the most liberal initial estimate provides.

Most new projects undertaken by People Places now include at least one and sometimes more initial meetings with upper- and mid-level agency staff regarding the operational components and resources essential to mounting an effective FFT program. We precede these contacts with monographs sent to key staff of the prospective client agency explaining the nature, background and supporting rational for foster family treatment as a program type (e.g., Bryant, 1980; Bryant, 1984; Snodgrass & Bryant, 1984). A primary goal in these pre-implementation efforts is to gain commitment from the client agency to what generally are seen as the core operational components of a sound foster family treatment program. These include low line worker caseloads (8 to 12), line worker expertise in applied behavior analysis and program planning, 24-hour on-call crisis intervention back-up, competency-based preservice treatment foster parent training, systematic use of the foster parent as an active agent of treatment, higher reimbursement rates to treatment foster parents, systematic in-home treatment programming and documentation for accountability (Bryant, 1980). We do not participate in development of a treatment foster care program unless a client agency is able to commit to fundamental program elements.

A one-day overview workshop is conducted by the People Places consultant during the pre-implementation stage of a typical program development project. The line and supervisory staff of the new program are joined in this workshop by upper-level agency administrators and other line and supervisory staff whose work may relate to or be impacted by the new program. If agency support for the new program is solid by this time, representatives from key human service agencies in the community are invited to the overview workshop. The purpose of the workshop is to fully describe the core elements of a foster family treatment program, People Places' technical assistance format, staff and parent training, and to secure the support of agency and community personnel throughout the hierarchy for each of these. A second overview workshop sometimes is held (often without the consultant's participation) to further articulate and sell the planned program internally or externally.

The core portion of the technical assistance model covers a period of six weeks and focuses on staff development, organization structure and process, and treatment foster parent training. The goals of this project stage are to make final specific policies and procedures for day-to-day operation, to train program staff in skills required to provide technical assistance to treatment foster parents focusing primarily on applied behavior analysis, in-home treatment program planning and social skills training methods, and to train the program's first group of prospective treatment foster parents.

Line and supervisory staff meet weekly for six weeks in three-hour afternoon workshops with the People Places consultant. The focus for the first two hours is on case study application and rehearsal of behavior analysis and program planning skills. The third hour of most sessions is devoted to organization planning and covers such operational issues as client selection, treatment foster parents recruitment, the pre-placement process, integration of out-of-home therapeutic services with the child's total program including individual/family counseling, relation with schools, reunification/ discharge planning, and program evaluation. These topic areas may vary somewhat from agency to agency depending upon local needs and orientation. Mid- and upper-level administrative staff are encouraged to participate in the organization planning hours of staff sessions. Staff from other units who may benefit from the treatment skills training are encouraged to join in all staff sessions to nurture their identification with and support for the new program and to spread the technical training as far as possible within the agency to help prepare for problems created by staff turnover.

The afternoon staff session is followed each week by a three-hour evening workshop for prospective treatment foster parents. The consultant leads participants through the six weekly sessions of parenting skills training. Local line, supervisory and training staff who will use the curriculum or provide in-home support to foster parents also attend evening session. In this way, the initial core group of treatment foster parents can be trained intensively while local staff learn to use the curriculum to train subsequent treatment foster parent groups. Staff-parent involvement in this initial sequence also serves an important team-building purpose. Mutual support, group cohesion and loyalty are developed along with concrete skills, all of which help sustain both parents and staff through what may be trying times during the new program's early months.

On-site follow-up by the consultant is available in addition to phone consultation available to all new program sites. Follow-up visits serve a technical purpose as modifications in the new program's operations nearly always are found necessary once youth have been placed and the program design has been tested under actual conditions. On-site follow-up visits also can serve an important motivational purpose both for parents and staff as the consultant typically is viewed as an ally as well as an expert. The format and content of on-site follow-up vary according to the needs of individual sites. Time is spent with staff and individual treatment foster parents reviewing and troubleshooting in-home teaching plans and designing plans for newly placed youth. Evening in-services support group meetings also have been organized around specific training topics and have been useful to encourage new foster parent applicants recruited by the original group of treatment foster parents.

This technical assistance model is the product of trial and error learning. Not all new programs require the intensity of assistance described here. For public agencies the creation of a new foster family treatment program represents a substantial political effort. In these agencies, more intensive and long-term technical assistance has been useful for program design and staff training and as a vehicle for securing broad and realistic support for the new program and the process of change its development requires.

PROGRAM DEVELOPMENT AT THE STATE LEVEL

Missouri's population of five million is found in both large urban areas (St. Louis and Kansas City) and relatively undeveloped, sparsely populated rural areas. The Missouri Department of Social Services Division of Family Services has responsibility for approximately 6500 children in alternate care. During recent years, the foster care population has declined and stabilized while the residential care population has grown rapidly.

The development of specialized foster care or foster family treatment by the Department began primarily as a result of external pressure and political considerations. In the early 1980s the situation with regard to residential care for youth had become critical; residential facilities were full and 250 and 300 youth were awaiting residential treatment while experiencing repeated disrupted placements in regular foster care. Pressure from child welfare advocates in the state for a resolution to this problem was mounting.

The Division director, one of 10 to hold the post over the previous 14 years, was beset with problems within the Division related to the lack of stable leadership during that time. In Jackson County (Kansas City area) criticism of foster care services had resulted in a federal consent decree whereby the local DFS was court-ordered to improve the quality of services to foster children and their caretakers. Pressure on the Division director translated to top level support for the development of foster family treatment programs around the state. Pressure on local agencies to provide placements for the growing number of youth referred to residential care likewise strengthened local interest in such programs. A perception was widely shared at state and local levels that many youth were placed inappropriately in residential care for lack of less restrictive treatment alternatives. The confluence of external and internal pressures for change provided a window of opportunity for developing a quality foster family-based alternative to residential care.

A 1984 conference provided an opportunity to discuss the concept of treatment foster family care with experts in the field and to begin to determine what would be required to develop pilot programs. Two state office staff were assigned to do further research and to assess the replicability of specific programs. We decided early on not to attempt to reinvent the wheel, but to adapt a proven model to our needs and circumstances. We used these criteria in selecting the program model to replicate in Missouri:

— The model program must have shown a history of growth and success.
— It must be based on the philosophy that foster parents are primary treatment agents and are an integral part of the professional team.
— The model program must provide an excellent, scripted training packet and related materials which would equip local staff to carry on with the program following initial training and consultation.
— Since we decided to contract for the initial treatment foster parent and staff training, we wanted consultants who had direct line experience in the field and could be realistic and have credibility with staff and foster parents.

People Places' program and training staff met all these criteria and a contract for technical assistance was awarded to them through a competitive bidding process.

The next step was to develop project sites. Our aim was to proceed at a measured pace so that a workable adaptation of the service model could be developed and sufficient time allowed to assess implementation at representative sites. We began with three sites—two urban and one rural. Our original plan was to select sites through a volunteer process, but we were faced with such political realities as the Jackson County consent decree, the need to include St. Louis if Kansas City (Jackson County) were selected, and the hesitance of local agencies statewide to take on any new program requiring commitment of additional time and resources. The first three pilot sites—Kansas City, St. Louis, and Joplin—were selected through a combined volunteer and pragmatic political process. In hindsight, a purely volunteer process, had it been possible, probably would have worked better by assuring stronger local administrative commitment in all areas.

We asked the administration at each pilot site to select staff and foster parents for the program and held orientation meetings with the staff chosen at each site. While this generally was a helpful strategy, our enthusiasm to sell the program caused one fairly serious complication. In describing the implementation plan, we suggested that resources would be made available to allow each site to contract with local clinicians who could provide ongoing consultation in behavioral programming and other therapeutic services, and that each site would be allocated an additional worker slot by the state office to allow for a lower caseload. Approval for these two components did not materialize as we had expected with the result that local project staff felt let down despite the substantial support and resources that were mobilized for program development.

In retrospect, we should have received clear written approval for all support elements we requested before sharing what we had asked for with local staff. Again, political pressures for timely implementation of the project and for a demonstration of the Division's commitment to action contributed to this mistake. Local commitment in two of the project sites was strong enough to overcome the initial disappointment regarding staffing and consultation. In both sites, means were found for assigning a reduced, specialized caseload to the line workers and for securing regular consultation from local behavioral psychologists. The third site responded to the project plan more as a directive than as an opportunity. The result was a weak commitment and program for the first year and a half of implementation.

We developed a draft program manual to provide broad policy and procedural guidelines to staff designing the local variations of the program. Flexibility and room for local initiative proved essential to successful program development. Each project site needed to adapt its program to local conditions both for practical purposes and to foster local agency buy-in to the project. The two sites which were most successful had mid-level managers who directly participated in all aspects of program development and adopted a whatever-it-takes view toward making the program work without compromising the core elements of the original service model. The program was less successfully implemented at a site which did not assign a direct supervisor to the project until after staff and parent training had been completed and did not provide a specialized worker to concentrate solely on a small caseload of special needs youth. These key components were added recently to that site's program, partly as a result of the momentum and initial success of other pilot sites developed around the state.

None of the project sites stayed fully within the program parameters defined originally by the state office. This occurred partly by design and partly by default. While the state office recognized the need for a degree of local autonomy, we did not have sufficient staff at the state level throughout the project period to allow for more rigid oversight even if that had been our intention. Local autonomy in designing and adapting a program suiting their needs proved positive in the two sites which stuck to the core program features. Where commitment to core service elements such as reduced worker caseloads was lacking, local autonomy undermined the development of a viable program. Allowing local staff to experiment and design their own program within a broadly stated framework resulted both in effective programs and greater local commitment.

PROGRAM DEVELOPMENT AT THE LOCAL LEVEL – KANSAS CITY

Kansas City was one of the three initial sites selected to pilot the treatment foster family program in Missouri. The agency is large, highly bureaucratized, and historically has been slow to enhance or expand the services it is mandated to provide. A court decree, however, directed the agency to provide needed training and increased services to foster parents and special needs youth in the area. Staff morale was adversely affected by the decree at the same time informal public and formal political and judicial pressures for change increased.

The first response when invited to participate in the project was to decline the offer. We thought the time allowed for foster parent recruitment and selling efforts with staff was insufficient for the task. When the invitation was restated in more directive terms by the state office, we had one month to select foster parents and prepare staff for staff and parent training. We did not apprise line and direct supervisory staff of our reservations but went ahead with preparations at a much accelerated rate.

Selling the project to line staff was not as difficult as might be imagined. Staff were well aware of the need for alternative placements for children with significant behavioral and emotional problems. Many actually had been encouraged by the recent court order to improve foster care services, hoping that additional resources would accompany the decree. Residential treatment centers were full, and there were no local funds remaining to place additional children in residential centers. Local staff greeted the program and the training which accompanied it with a generally positive and enthusiastic attitude. We had more trouble initially protecting the program from being inundated with referrals than we did with staff resistance.

A number of foster care staff were included in both staff and parent portions of the training. The project worker, several first- and second-level supervisors, one upper-mid-level supervisor, line staff from the regular foster care units and foster parent recruitment and licensing staff were all included in the training. There were several advantages to opening the training up in this way. First, a team spirit developed among staff participants which facilitated the project's acceptance within the agency and helped reduce any sense of isolation that the primary project worker might otherwise have felt. Second, supervisors learned the technical skills needed to assist the line worker and were prepared to train a new worker should that have become necessary. Other sites have experienced turnover in the worker position. Training other line staff and supervisors simultaneously is wise so that worker turnover does not have a terminal effect on the new program.

Broad guidelines were established by the state office regarding program policies and procedures. We modified some of these guidelines to make a better fit with local needs and conditions. For example, the state office originally specified that the program was to serve teenagers only. Locally, we had several very disturbed younger children who we felt could be diverted from institutional placement and provided a stable family placement through treatment foster care. The state was flexible in this and several other operational matters, which allowed us to customize the program to suit our needs without sacrificing program integrity. While local autonomy of this kind was helpful, guidelines should not be so flexible as to allow deviation from the core components of foster family treatment. In Kansas City, we freed a worker to specialize in foster family treatment and carry a much reduced caseload of eight to ten youth. In another project site, no single worker was designated for the program and foster family treatment cases simply were added to existing caseloads. This site did not experience the level of success that the two sites did which adhered to the fundamentals of the foster family treatment model as we learned it.

The program structure for foster family treatment can create problems as it is overlaid onto an existing system. The small caseload managed by the project line worker, while essential to effectiveness, occasionally is a source of resentment by other staff with large caseloads. Turf problems have arisen between regular foster care workers and home finders and the foster family treatment unit with regard to the use of homes. Early on, regular foster care workers placed children in trained treatment foster homes without the knowledge of the treatment foster care worker. Competition for scarce family resources, of course, is at the heart of this problem. Currently, any placements in a treatment foster home must be approved in advance by the treatment family worker, who seeks to minimize the number and disruptiveness of such additional placements. This may be resented since many of the children in regular foster care also exhibit behavior problems and have experienced several disrupted foster home placements. The resolution to this problem ultimately is beyond the means of our local agency and rests with decision makers who determine resource allocations for families and children.

The treatment foster care program is structured to allow for thorough assessment and matching. Workers referring children to the program have expressed some frustration at the amount of information we request concerning youth and at the amount of time required to complete placement. We do not place children on an emergency basis. A minimum of two separate overnight or weekend pre-placement visits to the prospective treatment foster home is required for all children placed to increase chances for a workable foster parent-child match.

HINDSIGHT: WHAT WE HAVE LEARNED

In hindsight, there are several things we would do differently in developing new foster family treatment programs.

We should have allowed more up-front time to recruit foster parents, prepare staff in all sites, and confirm precisely what resources would be available to each site in developing its program. In retrospect, we would have been wise to make our best estimate of the time required, then double it.

We used only experienced foster parents from within our current system to launch our program. While there were obvious advantages to this, some families already had children in their homes who could not rightly be moved simply because a child needing a treatment foster home was placed. Consequently, we faced administrative, supervisory and treatment problems from having traditional and treatment foster care combined in the same home and dealt with more children in some treatment foster homes than was optimal. We need to recruit from outside our current foster parent population from this program as well as from within.

A statewide initiative of this kind requires a full-time project coordinator. A new program requires ongoing technical assistance as well as daily communication between individual sites and the state office. A single central office coordinator could provide necessary support to localities, facilitate cross-fertilization among sites, and lobby more effectively at the state level for resources the localities need to sustain and expand successful efforts.

We should have designed and used a systematic evaluation process which could tell us how the program was doing as a whole and provide data which could help foster and advance administrative and legislative support. We need to document clearly that we are preventing more restrictive placements, that the youth we serve differ significantly from those in regular foster care, and that our program is cost-effective. While we do have some useful data on these issues and are now establishing a simple program evaluation process in the pilot sites, systematic collection of data from the start would have been preferable. Time constraints seemed to narrow our focus despite what we knew would be wise practice.

We should have assured that all local administrators as well as line and supervisory staff were enthusiastic initially and remained so throughout the implementation process. Enthusiasm remained high in two of the areas; in one, it did not. A this-too-shall-pass attitude at the local level can neither motivate nor sustain a difficult program development effort.

One site did not lower caseloads of project line staff to a maximum of eight to ten youth. We learned quickly that low caseloads are essential to allow for the intensive support and treatment planning/consultation foster parents need from line staff. Foster family treatment cannot be done by simply training staff and parents, then adding additional responsibilities to existing workloads. Local autonomy is helpful only where field staff have a strong understanding of and commitment to the program.

Expert technical assistance, while not magic, is helpful in developing a new program of this kind. Technical assistance was cost-effective for us by providing the tools and organizational design we would have spent considerably more time developing on our own. In hindsight, it is even more important than we originally understood to involve additional staff in the training both to broaden in-house support for the program and to prepare for later line worker turnover by having sufficient trained back-up staff.

Our experience in Missouri suggests that foster family treatment can be done by a large public agency. We at least know that viable programs can be developed and sustained on a pilot basis for two years. In 1987, we extended the program by adding four new sites. Each DFS administrative area in the state now has a pilot program in place serving youth who otherwise would be referred to residential care.

Despite some promising indications, however, we are at a critical juncture in Missouri with regard to foster family treatment. Our pilot phase seems to have been reasonably successful. To sustain the pilot programs and expand the model further, however, will require resources that may not be forthcoming. While we are learning that we can provide an alternative to many current residential placements through foster family treatment, we may not be able to implement such programs broadly and reduce costly institutional placements, because we do not have the dollars to mount the programs. One reason we do not have the dollars is that we are spending so much on residential placements. In short, we cannot afford to save. Sadly, what is lost in this dilemma is not dollars alone, but opportunities for normal living and learning experiences for children who need and deserve them.

It is early to claim that foster family treatment in Missouri is a success. We have begun a promising program and have gained a degree of respect and recognition from child welfare advocates, foster parents and local agency staff for our efforts and outcomes so far. The real challenge for us will be to obtain the solid commitment of resources needed to sustain and develop the program in the future.

Chapter 13

Group Therapy for Birth Parents of Children in Foster Care

Brian Charbonneau
Ziona Kaplan

ABSTRACT. Psychological impairments render many biological parents of children placed in treatment foster care incompetent to meet child-rearing tasks. Service agreements identify and address critical areas of dysfunctioning but do not engage parents in a broader inventory of their parental functioning and dysfunctioning. A group method provides mutual support, exploration, and a positive child-rearing model. A clinical assessment of parenting that highlights ongoing developmental needs of nurturance and empathy, limit setting, structure, role modeling, reality testing, and separation and individuation is used to promote progress. Parents gain insight into their own overall impairments, origin of impairments, and compensatory techniques. Parents recognize broader responsibility for parenthood enhancing reunification efforts.

INTRODUCTION

An increasing awareness that foster care is often a long-term, rather than short-term, solution has developed in the last decade (Fanshel & Shinn, 1978) resulting in concerted efforts to emphasize

Brian Charbonneau is Program Coordinator, and Ziona Kaplan is Clinical Social Worker at Child & Family Services, 1680 Albany Avenue, Hartford, CT 06105.

177

the importance of permanency planning in preventing foster care drift (Maluccio, Fein, Hamilton, Klier, Ward, 1980; Maluccio & Fein, 1983). A related change has been to expand the focus of attention to include the biological parents, as well as the children in care, when considering treatment plans. Public Law 96-272, the Adoption Assistance and Child Welfare Act of 1980, emphasized the responsibility of agencies to make reasonable efforts toward prevention of placements as well as toward family reunification when placement occurred. While reasonable efforts are not yet defined in practice, there remains the need to broaden treatment approaches to biological families.

Engagement and empowering of birth families whose children are placed in treatment foster care presents unique obstacles. This parent population has been characterized as "[They] . . . feel a sense of helplessness or powerlessness. They perceive themselves as victims of a system that controls them, and feel that they have no power over the decisions others are making about their lives and the lives of their children" (Maluccio, Fein & Olmstead, 1986, p. 145). Often birth parents have not recovered from their childhood traumas of neglect, abuse, or loss and are socially alienated. We will describe a program which has included group work for biological parents as part of its therapy for children in treatment foster care. It is a modest addition to a treatment foster care program, has resulted in handsome benefits, and requires neither wholesale changes in an existing program nor specially trained workers.

This group was established to more effectively outreach to isolated and difficult-to-treat birth parents by creating the opportunity to share and participate with similar families in a group setting. All of the parents needed help in learning and improving parenting skills. Learning together with other parents could produce additional benefits of a social and emotional nature.

The Specialized Foster Care Program at Child and Family Services provides permanency-planning-oriented, intensive, time-limited (one to two years) clinical treatment for the children and families. Often the children have experienced multiple placements. Their histories include emotional, physical, and sexual abuse; they may be aggressive, antisocial, withdrawn, isolated and/or developmentally delayed. Therapeutic foster families, a vital part of the treatment team, care for the children in close collaboration with the agency staff. Typically the child and biological family are seen weekly in individual and/or family sessions. Parent aides are available to help birth parents acquire parenting and household management skills. The ultimate goal is rehabilitation and reunification of both parents and children.

In 1984 we began a support group for the birth parents to provide social support, an introduction to parenting skills, and personal growth for members. This group meets weekly for one hour and ten minutes at the agency. The group is available to birth parents whose children are in care and reside in agency foster homes. Frequently the birth parents are involuntary clients who participate in their treatment regime to comply with court expectations. Birth parents in our program may reluctantly agree to a plan for therapy, but their expectation of frustration prevents them from being able to invest in a treatment alliance. The course of individual treatment is slow. At the same time we strive to decrease the length of out-of-home placement, so maximizing treatment efforts is critical.

Birth parents are unaccustomed to discussion of feelings and express confusion and decry the state and agency's forced therapy. Because their children have been placed against their will and are now being raised by other, supposedly better parents, the birth parents may experience strong anger and resentment about both their children's loss and their own involuntary therapy. Often these parents become involved to meet requirements for their child's return but may not be invested in the process for growth.

Although their children often make obvious gains, the birth parents do not seem to make corresponding progress except that they are more resentful than ever of the state intervention in their lives and, in some cases, more determined to keep to themselves permanently. The whole experience often seems more punitive than helpful.

The biological parents' lack of resources leads to limited treatment gains in individual therapy no matter how good the therapist. The sessions cannot be used for growth by the parents because they do not easily see the therapist as a helper who is interested in their growth. The parents are more likely to see the therapist as judgmental of both their poor parental attempts and lack of verbal skills. They are too isolated socially to realize that their problems are not particular to them alone and experience themselves as victims with little ability to alter the conditions in which they live or the outcome of events. This acute isolation and resentment against the therapist makes individual therapies sometimes unproductive for birth parents. Group therapy with parents is most beneficial because it eliminates the threatening one-on-one with the therapist, lessens the social isolation, allows a feeling of mastery as parents help each other learn parenting and self-respect, and provides a safe environment for parents to learn the rudiments of child development and personality theory so as to alter their negative world and child views.

GROUP METHODS

The elements of socialization, mutual support, and child-rearing education combine to make the birth parents group both unique and effective. The group begins with relaxed socializing time to help overcome timidity and fear that other people will discover lack of conversational and relating skills. The agency provides dinner for the parents and children they wish to invite. This purely social time is casual and provides families with opportunities for conversation with others. Each meeting begins with a joke and the understanding, however, that the following hour may touch on some difficult issues.

Parent Assessment Content

An hour is then spent in group discussion to enhance parents' capacity to provide nurturance and empathy, limit setting and structure, boundaries and roles, modeling, reality perceptions and individuation. These elements comprise a parenting assessment scale used in evaluating parental competency. By framing discussions, parents become familiar with these developmental elements, capable of rating themselves on a continuum, and able to identify their conflict areas as well as potentially more adaptive methods of relating to their children. Denial is lessened and ownership of problem areas accelerated.

The nurturance and empathy continuum refers to the parent's level of bonding and relatedness to the child. On the lower level of the continuum the parent is emotionally detached and profoundly self-serving; on the upper level the parent is able to respond with a steady mood state to the child and can ascribe value to the inner life of others regardless of the parent's own needs or environmental stressors. We discuss parents' abilities to put their children's needs before their own and focus on ways to enhance the children's self-esteem. The group is provided an explanation of the meanings of nurturance and empathy and how those exist as a basic need for children's development from the moment of birth. The symbol used over and over to stress its basic importance is the image of a bucket that continually needs filling. The question is raised concerning the parents' own buckets, and how is it possible for a bucket that feels empty to be able to fill someone else's (their child's). The bucket has become the metaphor for the parents' feeling state, one to which they easily relate, understand, and can use in assessing their child's emotional state and level of neediness.

Setting limits as a way to understand discipline for children is the next major point of emphasis. Limit setting means learning impulse control over one's aggression and frustrations. On the lower end of the continuum is the parent who is impulse-ridden, prone to outbursts of rage and able to totally rationalize acting on aggressive and sexual impulses; on the other end is the parent who is optimally self-controlled, sees shades of grey and is or can be both even-tempered and comfortable expressing anger. Our goal is to demonstrate that discipline is a way to help a child develop inner control of his or her behavior. Simply exerting control over a child by yelling, spanking, and threatening are ineffective in the long run because they promote more negative behaviors. Rewarding positive behaviors, emphasizing praise rather than criticism or punishment, offering logical consequences based on choices made by the child as opposed to orders imposed by parents are more productive and also more bucket-filling. A child's resistance to accepting limits is viewed as nascent self-boundary. Another aspect of limit setting is providing structure to family life; predictable routines and organization in family operation are important for encouraging healthy emotional growth for a child. Many of these parents have themselves grown up in disorganized-chaotic families where meals and bedtimes were never predictable, and they find themselves replicating a low structure model, with little understanding of how this ultimately impacts them and their children. Again, routines indirectly also fill the bucket.

Similarly, families are helped to understand the varying roles of each family member by seeing the structure of the couple, the parents, the siblings and how each subsystem acts within its own system, interacts between systems, and where the boundaries are set and how important it is to maintain them. Families who have clearer structure usually are more successful at establishing and maintaining the boundaries between subsystems and the activities within them.

The metaphor of a mirror is used to discuss modeling appropriate behavior, transmitting moral values, and showing how a parent's behavior is reflected in the child's behavior. Often parents are unaware of the degree to which children incorporate their parents' behaviors into their own. Parents in the group are asked to look at their own parents so as to recognize those similarities which they were unaware that they were now replicating. Parents are reminded that they are the ones who set the moral rules and are the role models to whom the children look for guidance in developing a healthy sense of right and wrong.

Reality testing refers to the level of accuracy in viewing objective events and ascribing subjective tones. At the lower end of this continuum are psychotic parents unable to distinguish inner from outer realities while the upper end reflects an ability to view events without prejudice, to distinguish the objective and subjective parts, and to be open to additional evidence. Parents need to promote a healthy reality perception of the events surrounding a child's life. Magical thinking and mistaken perceptions common to children's thinking are to be sorted out by objective-thinking parents.

The concept of separation-individuation leading to a level of self and object constancy and subsequently healthy object-relations in a developing child is presented in a simplified, jargon-free explanation. The idea is to help a child become his own person, separate from parent. This is a more sophisticated concept than the others, but one that becomes understandable through the use of real life examples and promotes insight into parents' own earlier experiences.

GROUP PROCESS

Repetition of the assessment elements provides parents with a cognitive tool for self-examination. Parents inquire, "Why do we find ourselves caught in this cycle of dysfunction?" and "How can we change to parent better than we were parented?" The group members are enlightened to learn how much they themselves, from their own neglected and deprived backgrounds, have been the victims. The cyclical nature of child-rearing and poor parenting is examined, the question of "Can we stop the cycle?" is raised and discussed.

One of the group leaders takes a particular problem, discussed by the group, to demonstrate the connection between that problem and one of the assessment elements. Often many weeks are spent examining one point and its many ramifications on parenting or family functioning. Role playing is used to point up an issue and to attempt to give families a method of learning and feeling. Another device is to ask group members to rate their own parents on a scale of one to ten and then themselves to look for similarities and unconscious influences. Handouts are presented or outlines are put on the blackboard. Parents take notes and are conscientious about learning. Most say they are learning a lot and at the same time they enjoy themselves. The atmosphere is relaxed and nonthreatening, and they feel safe asking questions or exposing their weaknesses.

Individuals use the group as support for the process of developing through their own treatment phases of the placement process. The group is an open-ended group where new members join and old ones leave depending on their place in their own placement period. As individuals, group members find that they experience an engagement phase, working-through phase, return of children phase (or termination of placement phase), and follow-up phase.

Initially many families feel reluctant to expose themselves to a group and feel threatened by taking the step to join. They feel embarrassed by the stigma of being seen as bad parents because their children have been placed in foster care. Their social skills are so underdeveloped that they feel inadequate to interact in a social milieu. They feel powerless against the authorities that seem to have taken over their lives, and they carry a deep reservoir of anger and resentment against the professionals who are attempting to help them. They often fear they will never get their children back. When they enter the room they meet others who are very much like themselves. They learn that they are not alone in any of their feelings or predicaments. They begin to hear hopeful, positive things from other members, such as favorable foster family stories, or news of impending return home of children. Individual participation begins to increase as members or couples become comfortable within the group. Often they look forward to presenting a problem they are struggling with at home and want group feedback. At this stage they are less defended and more open to criticism or advice, more willing to admit errors or mistakes. One mother wanted help in coping with a child telling outrageous lies. A father asked for suggestions on working with his child who has self-destructive temper tantrums. Group members offer feedback which will lead to a discussion of an underlying principle that has general application to all the group members. In the case of the child's lying, the group responded by pointing out the child's need for attention or possible anger at mother; members thought the temper tantrums were the result of inconsistent limit-setting by the father.

Learning that the period of placement is coming to a close and the child or children will be coming home is also a time of stress and ambivalence. Having a network of support during and following the termination of placement has proved to be invaluable. A single mother had had several emotional breakdowns and had not cared for her children for several years. She needed to complete her schooling, get a job, and find housing before they would be returned. All these goals were met; the children and she have been reunited for over a year, but she still attends group and says, "My children tell me I need to keep going to group because it keeps me honest!" Another mother stated when asked if she intended to continue coming after her son returned home, "Oh, of course I intend to continue with the group. After all, it's my only chance all week to have a social life!"

Where parental rights have been terminated, parents have been less able to make positive use of the group. Usually, these parents have suffered ego deficits too severe to repair or build up enough self-esteem to allow them adequate emotional strength to resume a parental role. Some have made an effort to participate in the group experience for a time but they were unable to sustain the work towards reunification.

DISCUSSION

Birth parent treatment is a valuable adjunct to the repertoire of permanency planning services focused on family rehabilitation and reunification. Parents benefit from the group experience in a number of ways. The sense of community established in sharing their struggles with one another affects their self-esteem positively; they are engaged in mutual support and become more invested in the opportunity for clinical services. They secure a framework to think about and discuss themselves and their children. The birth parents' commitment to improving their parenting skills becomes incorporated into their lives for their own and their children's sake rather than limited to the period of the court's intervention. The pace of individual and/or family treatment is accelerated, and voluntary post-reunification services are often requested by families. Once a parent experiences competence as a group member – both receiving and offering support and guidance – the array of community-based self-help groups such as Parents' Anonymous become available. Agency based fee for services too are more likely to be sought. A birth parent group extends the range of services supporting family integrity. The foster care service substantially increases its therapeutic presence at relatively minimal cost.

Chapter 14

Foster Care:
Last Resort
or Treatment of Choice?

Ziona Kaplan
Edith Fein

ABSTRACT. Specialist foster family care may be the treatment of choice for emotionally disturbed or behaviorally unmanageable children. The child and family often need a break and breathing space from each other. The child and birth parents can be involved in a treatment group, and the foster parents will be seen regularly so they may be involved in supporting the treatment goals. Biological parents will benefit from observing the foster family as role models in parenting, and practitioners are able to examine and reinforce the coping and adapting skills of the children.

How do workers, families or other referring sources determine where to place a troubled child from a troubled family? The trend is to make every effort to keep families together, a high priority of the permanency planning movement. Permanency planning addresses concern that children's growth and development is impaired by instability, uncertainty, and longevity of a child's experience with a temporary and remedial placement program. Various in-home interventions have been proposed including parent-aides (Miller, Fein, Howe, Gaudio, & Bishop, 1984) and outpatient family therapy

Ziona Kaplan is a Clinical Social Worker at Child and Family Services, 1680 Albany Ave, Hartford, CT 06105. Edith Fein is Director of Research at Casey Family Program East, 36 Woodland Street, Hartford, CT 06106.

(Kerr, 1981). Sometimes the very thing the family may need, however, is the dreaded disruption (Kirgan, 1983). The child and family may well need a break and breathing space away from each other. Specialized foster care placement is often not only an appropriate option but may be the best possible choice.

The Specialized Foster Care (SFC) offered by Child & Family Services, Hartford, Connecticut, is structured from the outset to be time-limited (1-2 years), provides foster families trained to offer therapeutic environments for troubled children, and provides intensive services within a prescribed time frame to arrive at a permanent plan for each child. The child is seen weekly for therapy; the foster family is seen weekly to discuss ongoing issues and progress of the child; whenever possible the biological parents are seen for therapy and counseling so they can participate in the rehabilitation and decision-making process; and social workers have small case loads to allow for adequate time for each case.

What are the considerations for SFC placement? Children referred to this program are presented as emotionally disturbed or behaviorally unmanageable. Often they have had several foster home disruptions before turning to a SFC option. Interactions between the child and birth family have reached a point where they appear to be unable to coexist under the same roof. After assessing the presenting needs of the child and the family, the SFC social worker attempts to match a foster family to the child. The choice of a SFC home for particular children from dysfunctioning family systems has been shown at times to produce amazing results. We can sometimes create situations where the intervention of foster placement and the child's apparently hidden ego strengths have enabled the child to adapt readily to the new family and has afforded such vast relief for the child that changes are able to occur rapidly. Some children who have been presented as so severely disturbed that they could be considered candidates for a more restrictive setting, such as a residential or hospital facility, were found to improve rapidly — emotionally, behaviorally, and cognitively.

Shortly after placement the child may quickly lose symptoms and begin to demonstrate adequate ability and functioning. This raises eyebrows among foster parents and professionals alike. What happened to this disturbed child? Was this child not as troubled as professionals had assessed? Was the child merely reflecting the disturbance in his own family by limitation, identification, adaptability, or assignment of role by other family members? Two case examples will illustrate this phenomenon.

THE CASE OF CLARA

This referral came from a local children's hospital. Clara Sandstone was four and a half years old, small in stature, immature and delayed in her behavioral development, cognitively deficient having tested at a retarded level, emotionally deprived, and she also suffered from partial hearing loss. Her diagnosis was atypical developmental disorder or psycho-social dwarfism; she was considered developmentally and physically delayed and severely disturbed.

Her parents presented difficulties. The father, Mr. Sandstone, was apparently of low cognitive functioning. He spoke in a dull, limited way and was completely dependent for approval on his wife. There was a child-like quality in his relationship with her. Mrs. Sandstone seemed to be in charge of their relationship completely; she was of normal intelligence but was highly rigid, obsessional, anorexic, and narcissistic. Much of her ritualized, obsessional behavior was being transmitted to Clara so that Clara behaviorally reflected many of her mother's behavioral concerns. For example, she worried about food, what she could and could not eat, and she was obsessive in bathroom needs, elimination and vomiting. Mrs. Sandstone was incapable of nurturing the child and most of her interactions with Clara were rejecting in nature.

Clara's biological parents were only functioning marginally, barely adequately even for themselves, and the additional pressure of raising a child was overwhelming to them. They had inadvertently or unconsciously squelched Clara's growth; a baby in a crib was less frightening than a growing, developing child. Mrs. Sandstone had been married previously, produced a child from that union, was later divorced, and the child was in the custody of her father. The hospital staff determined that Clara was at risk remaining at home with her parents. Mrs. Sandstone was too obsessional and paranoid to allow parent aide services and Clara was at too great a risk to remain at home. Foster care, with the intention of offering intensive, rehabilitative therapy to the parents, was recommended. The task for the therapist was to recognize the needs of the parents and to understand that they needed help and permission to give up their child without feeling guilt, for both their own sakes and for that of their daughter. They needed to feel they were not bad parents, but were instead doing for their daughter what she most needed. This was not a simple task because they were ambivalent and confused, and the public agency workers had initially encouraged them to plan for Clara's return home.

Clara was placed with Mr. and Mrs. David, both of whom were available almost full-time to their children. The Davids had a grown family of five and now had a second family of two adopted girls. Mrs. David was interested in making a serious commitment to work with a troubled child. Both Mr. and Mrs. David were able and eager to offer Clara love, affection, encouragement, acceptance, learning, experience, social interactions, and physical play.

Clara experienced fitful sleeping habits, night crying, speech articulation problems, borderline echolalia, insecurity, and separation anxiety early in the placement. She left the table several times during meals to eliminate and talked regularly about elimination needs. She appeared to be highly stressed and anxious. With a good high protein diet, reassurance during night crying, touching, teaching, and consistently being told she was loved, Clara began to relax, trust the Davids, and become aware that she could control her life. As she was offered choices the stress decreased. She gradually became accustomed to a new world that was less rigid and pressured and more benign and accepting; her inappropriate behaviorisms decreased. Her hearing problems, which were discovered to be real, were also ameliorated by insertion of peditubes in her ears.

Clara began to show interest in learning and experiencing the larger world around her. She had been confined to a dark dingy apartment in an urban area, never allowed out to play, often confined to bed, and forced to watch endless hours of television. Now Clara voraciously lapped up the generous amounts of food and a generous offering of affection and acceptance. Mrs. David spent time with her each day reading books and helping Clara recognize words and symbols commonly known to all four and a half year olds. Clara spent time learning basic motor skills such as running, jumping, tricycle riding, and swimming. She related well to her foster siblings, quickly gained weight, and grew inches seemingly overnight. She was attaching herself to the Davids and becoming a normal family member, full of life and spirit, love, and intelligence. Her potential in all areas now seemed high, and she was being considered a bright child.

THE CASE OF ROB

Rob, a ten-year-old, was referred because his mother had been looking for a possible residential placement for him. Rob's behavior with his birth family was so oppositional and charged with physical aggression, rage, and frustration, that he appeared to be on the verge of a breakdown. Life at home was intolerable for him and his family.

He was the older of two sons in a single-parent family. His parents had been divorced for six years and Rob and his brother lived at home with their mother in a house owned by her parents, who lived next door. The grandparents were elderly and in need of some physical assistance and supervision, but they had not relinquished their authoritarian role over their daughter and her children. Mrs. Baldwin, Rob's mother, was caught up in an extended family system with blurred boundaries and enmeshed emotions. Mrs. Baldwin had no confidence in her parenting ability, was treated like a child by her own mother, and treated like a peer by Rob. Rob, who was bright, constantly debated with her, was engaged in power struggles that he usually won, and as a result he usually felt guilty or angry.

Foster placement was suggested because the family issues were too intensive for parent aide intervention. Rob was petrified at the idea of leaving his family and moving to a strange new place although part of him was yearning to be free of the tensions and worries of his family. The placement with the foster family was carefully worked out, allowing Rob ample opportunity to know and feel comfortable with the Fairmont family.

The Fairmont foster family appeared to be just what Rob needed. The foster mother was a woman who knew her role, felt relaxed, and was in charge of her family. The father and other children in the home also had clear senses of identity, roles, and boundaries. The parents were the parents; the children knew, accepted, and respected this, so that the entire atmosphere was clear-cut and relaxed. Rob's adjustment, to everyone's surprise, was rapid. It appeared that Rob's main feeling was relief. His tension, fear, rage, and aggression seemed to quickly dissipate. Rob discovered that he was functioning normally, an important insight, because secretly he had feared for a long time that he was crazy.

Anger at his father, who he felt had abandoned him, was one of the first issues addressed in his therapy sessions. The worker suggested attempting to locate his father and writing him a letter. Much time was spent composing the letter, initially suggested by the social worker as "what you would like to say to your dad if you ever had the opportunity." After working together with Rob in the hypothetical letter to express what Rob really felt about his dad, the worker asked how he would feel about actually mailing the letter. He was all for it, even knowing that he might not get an answer. As it happened, his father did respond, a visit was subsequently arranged, and a new relationship was established between them. This helped him a great deal to let go of much of his pent-up anger.

Another element in therapy was helping mother and son redefine themselves and their roles within the family. Mrs. Baldwin needed support for assuming her role as an adult child of her parents and parent to her own children. Rob needed to be reminded that he was 10 and that he was not responsible for taking care of his mother. He needed permission to allow himself to be a kid and concern himself with kid's concerns. This realization helped greatly to lower his anxiety and tension. His behavior had been typical of many older sons of single parents who often unconsciously assume the burden of husband. Mrs. Baldwin had been suffering financial deprivation since her divorce, was unable to find good employment, and was dependent on her parents for her home and for babysitting. Her social life and social supports were minimal; she had a need to be worried, concerned, and involved with her children as a way of distracting herself from her own underlying depression. Rob's problems and her fears of the younger boy's growing problems were a consequence of her need to have that defense.

CASE OUTCOMES

A year and a half of therapy for both Mrs. Baldwin and Rob, though by no means successfully breaking their patterns of interaction, at least helped them both to know and understand how they affected one another. Rob and his mother made gains in separating and individuating themselves, setting up stronger boundaries, and defining their roles. These gains helped to break down their fused, enmeshed family interactions. When Rob returned home, both he and his mother were armed with new insights and improved coping skills, both were able to benefit from increased awareness.

Clara continued to progress in all areas of her life. She developed a positive self-image, a sense of humor, and an awareness of and sensitivity to others in a very caring way. When initially placed she required a great deal of sleep, inappropriate for her age, but as she grew to her normal size and physical growth, she leveled off to 11-12 hours at night with no daytime nap. Gymnastics classes helped her develop her motor skills and social interactions. Clara's mother's guilt over not being able to cope with parenthood had resulted in her labelling the child weird and retarded. She claimed mental retardation ran in her husband's family. Clara was called environmentally disadvantaged, learning disabled, and severely disturbed, and was well on her way to fulfilling the prophecy by becoming an institutionalized child. Her bizarre behavior, bland stares, and lack of comprehension were partly the result of a thirty percent hearing loss in both ears which was not attended to until foster placement. In the end, with the support and guidance of the SFC social worker and the public agency workers, Clara's parents voluntarily terminated their parental rights and she became free for adoption. The Davids were delighted to be able to make Clara a permanent member of their family.

These are both examples of the best practical application of the permanency planning theory, using creative solutions and considering ecological implications. One can invoke family systems theory to explain the dynamics of these cases and outcomes. To the degree that a family system is healthy, the degree of health of its members emerge (Kerr, 1981, pp. 234-235). Systems thinking does not look for the cause within the individual. In contrast, systems theory conceptualizes the appearance of a symptom as reflecting an acute and/ or chronic disturbance in the balance of emotional forces in that individual's important relationship systems, especially the family system.

The use of specialized foster family care may be the service of choice when a child's behavior is so dysfunctional that he or she cannot be managed in regular foster care or with an in-home parent aide, where biological parents may benefit from observing a foster family as role models in parenting, or where practitioners need to examine and reinforce the inherent coping and adaptive skills of children. The SFC program responds to behavioral problems as symptoms of a child's effort to have needs met rather than classifying and labelling the child.

PART III:
PROGRAM APPROACHES

Chapter 15

Therapeutic Foster Homes
for Teenage Mothers and Their Babies

Grace W. Sisto
Myra C. Maker

ABSTRACT. The Children's Aid and Adoption Society of New Jersey developed therapeutic foster homes for young mothers and their babies in response to the complex problem of teenage out-of-wedlock childbearing. The program assesses parenting capabilities and helps the mother make an early and informed decision regarding permanency for her baby. A full range of support services are offered the mother to test her decision to keep her baby under favorable conditions.

AGENCY BACKGROUND

The Children's Aid and Adoption Society (CAAS), established in 1899 as a private nonsectarian society, was founded by commu-

---

Grace W. Sisto is Executive Director, and Myra C. Maker is Clinical Supervisor at Children's Aid & Adoption Society of New Jersey, 360 Larch Avenue, Bogota, NJ 07603.

nity leaders who were concerned about dependent, neglected, abandoned, and abused children. It is a nonprofit corporation governed by a thirty-member board comprised of private citizens. The staff includes professionally trained caseworkers and consultants in allied fields. The CAAS umbrella covers many programs, all dedicated to improving the quality of life for children and the ability of families to deal with the problems they face in today's world. CAAS services include adoption, day care, foster care, and adolescent residential programs. Adolescents in care may be placed either in one of our group homes or with a treatment foster family. They can be moved between these services to assure that the program provided is always the one that serves the best interests of the child.

The CAAS Treatment Homes (TH) Program was developed in 1975 as an alternative approach to treating emotionally disturbed adolescents who require residential therapeutic services. In this program foster parents are recruited and trained to deal with the youths' specific emotional and behavioral problems. This service is provided under a contract with the New Jersey Division of Youth and Family Services (DYFS) for the placement of 28 youth including pregnant teenagers and unwed mothers and their infants. The TH Program was developed to broaden the agency's adolescent treatment capability by offering alternative options for children needing therapeutic services. The mission of the Treatment Homes Program is to help youth assigned to our care reach their best potential. Treatment Home parents must have a basic belief in the possibility for growth and development but also a recognition that problems arise from a combination of biosocial factors. Foster families are recruited, trained, and supervised by the agency professional staff. They agree to learn the skills needed to deal with the youth's specific emotional and behavioral problems and provide support at every step of the journey towards a productive life. In 1983, mother and child pairs were added to the core program and families were recruited to care for them to help them become adequate parents to their children. The young women selected for this program are under 22 years of age, have no family resources, and have been identified as socially or emotionally maladjusted.

THE PROBLEM

According to a 1983 study by the Alan Guttmacher Institute, the pregnancy rate for Americans 15 to 19 years old stands at 96 per 1,000, compared with 14 per 1,000 in the Netherlands, 35 in Sweden, 43 in France, 44 in Canada, and 45 in England and Wales. The level of sexual activity was reported to be about the same in the western countries cited (Jones, et al., 1985). The out-of-wedlock statistics in New Jersey in 1985 reported almost ninety-nine thousand cases, with approximately four thousand under 18 years of age.

Teenage childbearing is associated with adverse, pervasive, and long-lasting social and economic consequences for young parents, especially adolescent mothers, who at very young ages also appear to be at a higher risk of maternal morbidity and mortality (Chilman, 1980). Many children born to teenagers suffer intellectual deficits, largely because of the economic and social impact of early childbearing on young parents. Such children are more likely to spend part of their childhood in one-parent households and to have children themselves while still adolescents (Baldwin and Cain, 1980; Armstrong, 1981).

Many of these teenage mothers have no family support systems on which to rely. They are young women with serious educational deficits, no funds, and child responsibilities for which they are ill equipped. The Division of Youth and Family Services (DYFS) in New Jersey has been placing young mothers and their babies in separate foster homes. This is certainly the least desirable arrangement since the mother who has elected to keep her baby is separated from the child. The teaching of parenting skills or an assessment of her parenting capabilities cannot be accomplished at a distance. The child's attachment to the foster parent is an additional complication.

PROGRAM DESCRIPTION

The program goal is to develop therapeutic treatment homes for teenage unwed mothers who elect to keep their babies, to prepare the mother for independent living and parenthood, and to provide the baby with a safe, supervised, consistent environment during this period. The infant's future welfare can best be protected by an early permanent placement decision. This supervisory and assessment period is intended to test the mother's motivation and permit the treatment team to evaluate the mother's decision to keep her baby.

The adolescent mother is required to complete her education or attend a vocational training program during the period of foster care. She is expected to assume full responsibility for her infant when not in attendance at a program. The baby is enrolled in the CAAS Child Development Center from 8:30 to 5:30, Monday through Friday. In this arrangement, the young mother is relieved of primary responsibility for her child during her school or training program hours. She is required to spend some time at the day care center participating in the program with her infant under professional supervision. The mother benefits from the training she receives and from staff assessment of the dynamics of the relationship between the mother and child.

The enrollment of the child in the day care program may span 5 years, continuing after the mother's discharge from the TH program. This is a critical aspect of the design because it permits ongoing supervision during the child's important formative preschool years. Regularly scheduled parent group sessions help the young mother develop a support system to mitigate against feelings of isolation and depression. Counseling and other support services continue to be available during the entire 5-year period.

The TH couples or single adults recruited for this program are trained and supervised by CAAS professional staff and paid a fee for their services and a monthly board rate for the mother and child. They are considered staff workers with all the responsibilities this implies. They are expected not only to model parenting and home management skills but, over a specific time period, to help assess the parenting capabilities of the young mother. The TH parent thus becomes the support person in the home for both mother and child, being careful not to replace the mother as the parent.

The ultimate goals of this project are (1) to assess parenting capabilities in a supportive environment and encourage an early and informed decision regarding a permanent plan for the infant; (2) to discourage dependency on the welfare system by preparing the mother for an independent role as a parent and wage earner; and (3) the prevention of child abuse. The service is designed to support the mother through this transition period as well as afterward. The support team consists of the TH parent, the agency social workers, and the program consultant. Adoption counseling is initiated if it is determined after careful case management that the mother is incapable of parenting the child and the child would be at risk if discharged into the mother's care. A petition for the termination of parental rights would be used as a last resort.

Treatment Homes

In order for parents to become treatment parents, essentially to convert their home into a residential treatment center, CAAS provides significant services. Each family receives a home study in which they have the opportunity to consider the step they are taking and its effect on the family. CAAS, in turn, evaluates the family's capacity to care for difficult children. Mutual decisions can be made about what kinds of children and problems the family is best equipped to help.

After parents are approved for the program, and before a child is placed with them, they will begin to work together in a group consisting of other participating parents and the CAAS staff. The group meets every other week for approximately two hours to communicate, share knowledge, and develop treatment plans for individual children. The development of the skills necessary for the difficult task of treating the youth is the work of this group. The TH parents are expected to attend, and a portion of their fee is payment for their attendance. The purpose of the group meeting is to make the most of every opportunity for the youth's growth and development, and to discuss each youth's special needs.

The TH parent is responsible for all decisions made within the home, and the youth must respect this authority. If the youth senses that the parents are uncertain, or if there are no clear house rules, she may try to manipulate the parents. Youth must abide by a curfew that is set by the TH parents and other reasonable rules that the family feels are important to maintain order in the home. Each family has the opportunity to review referral information to determine if they will be able to work with a particular girl. Every effort is made to place the right girl with a family considering age, sex, ethnic background or race, family make-up, and most especially the girl's personality and particular problems.

Weekly contact, almost always a home visit, is made with each treatment family to deal with ongoing problems, to prevent problems, deal with crises, and to support the families in the difficult work they are doing. Families have 24-hour access to the program social workers for emergencies. The social worker also has a therapeutic relationship with the youth in placement. Support services for the youth in care are developed by the social worker and TH family. These include psychotherapy, special education services, medical and dental care and recreational activities. Available services in the community are used and all mental and physical health care is covered by Medicaid. The program is intended to extend for an 18-month period; however, this is a useful contracting device and not a fixed period of time. The controlling factors in determining length of placement are the teenager's need for this type of care and the capacity of the TH family to provide it. Discharge from the program is hopefully by plan but may occur any time that the youth cannot be maintained in an open community and family setting. If a girl has violated the law or presents dangerous behavior, removal can be effected quickly. In circumstances where the situation is deteriorating but not dangerous, CAAS send a 30-day report to the state department who will remove a youth within that period. However, girls may be placed in one of our group homes if the family requests immediate removal.

Accountability Requirements

An evaluation clinic is held biweekly to review the teenager's progress. Each case is scheduled for staff discussion 30 days after placement, and then quarterly throughout their stay in the program. The treatment parents, the program social workers, the girl's DYFS worker, the director of adolescent services, the clinical supervisor, and the program psychologist attend these meetings.

The social worker assigned to the girl presents a written progress report documenting the background, behavior this quarter, relationships, family issues, education, therapy, vocational and recreational activities of the youth. The treatment team then discusses the report and determines a treatment plan containing clear, specific, and operational recommendations in each category, i.e., what will be done, by whom, and in what time frame. CAAS also schedules an internal review meeting for each youth three months after placement and every six months thereafter to assess case progress. Attending this meeting are the program social workers, supervisory staff, as well as the executive director. This internal review committee is the permanency planning body of the agency, meeting to assure that each child needs to continue in care and that the short- and long-term goals are being addressed as stated in the treatment plan.

If any unusual incident occurs such as an accident, act of violence, runaway psychiatric emergency, or involvement with police or school authorities over illegal behavior, an incident report is written for the file and sent to the DYFS worker. Copies of all incident reports are given to the Executive Director, Clinical Supervisor, and Director of Adolescent Services within 24 hours of the occurrence. This allows members of the team to keep apprised of any unusual events in the youth's life.

The TH caseworker is the advocate for the family as a unit and is responsible for case management and implementation of treatment plans for the youth. This includes regular contacts with the girl, the TH parents, the girl's biological family if one exists, and participation in group meetings. The caseworker and the TH parents work together to obtain services, arrange family visitors, therapy, and other appointments that the youth requires.

PROGRAM IMPLEMENTATION

DYFS encouraged and financially supported this program design, and a contract was signed on April 1, 1983 for a pilot study. An important feature of this design is the payment of a fee of $500 plus a board rate for each month that the home is occupied. A separate stipend is paid to the young mother for the care of her infant. The TH parents monitor this latter fund. Two well-written editorials in local newspapers resulted in a large number of highly qualified applicants. The mature, professional people who responded led us to believe that the applicants viewed their role in this program as teachers or counselors and not as typical foster parents. Many of the applicants were social workers or in allied professions. After the initial phase, the program did not receive as many applicants but many of those who responded proved to be highly competent and receptive to skills training.

Many case referrals were received from DYFS and homes filled quickly. First experiences indicated that the program goals were being met successfully and that the design promoted early and informed decision making on the part of the young parent. Two mothers out of the four initially admitted to the program, for example, bonded well with their infants and the support services offered had a motivating influence on their behavior. The other two mothers were preoccupied with being adolescents at the expense of their infants. They resisted caring for their babies at the Child Development Center. The TH parents carefully logged the mother's impatience, lack of attention to proper feeding, and general irritability with their infants. The program requirements that the mother assume full responsibility for her baby when not attending her own program proved too much for these young mothers and these cases moved in the direction of eventual relinquishment for adoption placement.

One particular problem encountered early in the program was the large number of inappropriate referrals received from DYFS. The program was designed to work with mothers who have some potential for parenthood. Many of the young girls referred, however, were under 15 years of age and/or seriously mentally handicapped. These young women were not capable of assuming parental responsibilities and no pretense should be made in this direction. They should be referred to permanent planning units. Extended family resources might be sought to assist them or adoption counseling should be initiated as early as possible to help them relinquish the child.

The common problem areas of unwed mothers include:

1. Lack of positive self-identity.
2. Lack of ability to plan for the future or to delay gratification.

3. Lack of trust of caretakers.
4. Lack of positive experiences with initiative and autonomy resulting in poor work achievement and self-discipline (Vincent, 1961).

The Mother/Child Program addresses each of these points and attempts to mitigate against these influences. Admitting a teen parent into this special and selective program gives her the message that others have confidence in her potential; that she is so worthwhile that time, energies, and funds are being invested in her with the intent of promoting a more positive self-image. The young mother is now given guidance and can better tolerate frustration and the postponement of gratification. Her social workers and, most importantly, her TH parents, patiently and gently teach her the immediate consequences of behaviors and the future implications of these behaviors. Perhaps for the first time in her life the adolescent experiences a positive relationship with a parental figure developing a sense of trust in others. The TH parent constantly sets up win situations for the girl so that gradually and experientially she learns how to take care of herself and her child and even derives satisfaction from this newfound sense of autonomy.

The strengths of the Mother/Child Program are in providing security, guidance, nurturance, and opportunities for achievement, based on the assumption that this mother is a worthwhile human being. The girls are encouraged to finish school, to develop a marketable skill, to be independent of the welfare system, and to value their babies as much as they were made to feel valued in this program. Even if specific girls cannot attain these goals, the program helps them to do what is best for themselves and their children by giving them the opportunities for a timely assessment of their parenting potential and for counseling around seeking other options.

Chapter 16

PATH:
Putting Foster Parents in Charge

Michael Peterson

ABSTRACT. Established in 1972 in Minnesota, the PATH program is relatively unique in being a foster parent membership organization in which foster parents elect a board of directors responsible for establishing agency policies. Seven characteristics of the program are the central role of foster parents, individually developed treatment, goal orientation, close foster parent-social worker relationship, educational support, network of support relationships, and professional expectations.

Path was founded in 1972 in Minnesota to provide an alternative model for delivery of foster care (Galaway, 1976, 1978). The agency is a membership organization; all PATH foster parents are members of the nonprofit corporation and elect a board of directors which establishes policies and determines who to employ. Thus PATH is a foster parent-governed agency. An organization like PATH raises two questions: Can foster parents actually successfully govern an agency? If so, what kind of agency would they create?

The first question is answered by PATH's existence. The agency has survived and grown for fifteen years and is currently serving 195 children in 110 homes from offices in four areas of Minnesota. The annual budget is about 2.5 million dollars secured solely from fees for services; PATH has never needed to raise outside funds for

Michael Peterson is Executive Director of PATH (Professional Association of Treatment Homes), 1730 Clifton Place, Minneapolis, MN 55403.

operations. The PATH service model has been followed by a number of public and private foster care programs in Minnesota and other states. PATH's fifteen years of growth and stability demonstrate that foster parents can successfully govern an agency.

The answer to the second question is that they have developed a foster family-based treatment program in which the treatment is provided in a foster family rather than a group home, residential treatment center, or the child's own home. PATH programming emphasizes the development and maintenance of strong healthy foster families in which the foster child can heal and grow. The child benefits from the modeling in the home, the nurturing and teaching of the foster parents, and the counseling and treatment provided by all the members of the treatment team. PATH is not unique in providing foster family-based treatment. Other agencies have revised and improved on some aspects of the PATH model; these improvements have been looped back to help the PATH board and employees improve its programs. Thus an interchange of ideas has resulted in several Minnesota agencies following similar practices. These agencies and their common practices constitute the Minnesota model of treatment foster care. There are seven basic characteristics of the model.

CENTRAL ROLE OF FOSTER PARENTS

The PATH program is foster parent-centered. This means that agency social workers and administrative services are organized around supporting foster parents. The central role of foster parents means that foster parents are the primary treatment providers. The foster parents provide the primary help to the child in care. A treatment team is developed to assist the foster parents in working with each child. This team includes natural parents, referring social workers, teachers, counselors, therapists, and the PATH social worker. Successful teams work with and through the foster parents. The parents are the core of the team, with the foster child and birth family being the primary client. Other team members must recognize the need to work through the parents to serve the client.

INDIVIDUALLY DEVELOPED TREATMENT

PATH does not have a unitary approach to be followed with every child. Instead, the team endeavors to develop individual programs to meet the needs of each child. Efforts are made at placement to match the special needs of the child with the special strengths of the foster family. An individual treatment plan is developed for each child during the placement process. Each plan specifies the goals of the placement and the responsibility of the different team members and is developed at a planning meeting involving all the team members. The PATH social worker leads the meeting and writes the agreement which is signed by all members. PATH has 195 children and youth in care and 195 different treatment programs with individual treatment plans for each child. The point is to not have each foster family learn and follow the same approach, but rather to identify and enhance the skills of the foster parents at meeting the special needs of a specific child.

GOAL ORIENTATION

The treatment plan is based on clearly defined goals so that team members understand what they are trying to accomplish. One foster parent who had come from a regular foster care program described PATH as "foster care with a purpose." Joint goal setting is important for foster parents who otherwise may feel like pawns in someone else's treatment design for the child. Most human service professionals will agree that treatment goals are important; foster care, however, requires clearly understood goals written from the perspective of foster parents. When goals are clear, roles and responsibilities also become clear, ensuring that individual team members know what they are doing and why.

CLOSE FOSTER PARENT-
SOCIAL WORKER RELATIONSHIP

Foster parents and social workers maintain close working relationships. The relationship is developed through regular consultation and discussion and serves as the primary education and support for foster parents. The foster parent has the same social worker through all phases of the program. This includes licensing, relicensing, placements, and the services to each child in placement. Foster parents also will have the same social worker facilitating their support group meetings and working with the other families in their unit.

The social workers' primary responsibility is to provide assistance and support to the foster parents, to hold the foster family together so that the foster parents are able to provide services to the child. The social worker is educator, booster, counselor, and occasionally a shoulder to cry on for foster parents. The social worker also is responsible for liaison activities with other professionals such as therapists or referring social workers. To do this well requires small social work caseloads. The PATH foster parent board has established a policy that no social worker caseload will have more than 20 children. The average caseload is 15. Foster parents also recognize the importance of attracting qualified social workers. PATH social workers must have a master's degree or ten years of experience to be considered for employment. Salaries are ten to twenty-five percent higher than average social work salaries in the state. PATH parents want workers to be skilled in their services, professional in demeanor, and available for emergencies. The social worker job is arranged to meet the needs of foster parents; a nine-to-five approach does not work. The PATH social work salary is based in part on the number of children on the caseload rather than hours or days worked. Foster parents do not need social workers to work 40 hours; instead they need social workers to do whatever is needed to meet the needs of the children in placement.

EDUCATIONAL SUPPORT

Foster parents are provided opportunities for professional education through social worker-foster parent interaction, participation in support group meetings, PATH-sponsored training workshops, and individual education. The last three involve formalized training. Each foster parent must receive at least 30 hours of formal training each year. PATH directly provides at least 30 hours in each area of the state.

In addition, each foster family has $400 per year to purchase individual education. Education based on individual needs and interests is important, since the program is designed to meet individual needs of foster children.

The foster parent board has said that education is important enough that they will pay for it. Two years ago the PATH members had an opportunity to raise their rates but chose not to do this, and instead the board voted to put the money into education. The foster parents want quality courses so that they can better serve children and want individual education allowances so that they can address individual learning needs.

NETWORK OF SUPPORT RELATIONSHIPS

PATH creates an environment that is supportive of foster parents who work with difficult children and families. Effective support must be provided at a variety of levels. Support groups in which participation is required are a crucial part of the PATH support program. PATH foster parents are divided into units of 5 to 10 families. These units meet as the support group. The meetings become combination clinical staffing and sharing time. The group members sustain and encourage each other as they discuss the children in care and give each other a wealth of practical suggestions for dealing with daily behaviors. The foster parents develop friendships which benefit them outside of the meeting. The social workers facilitate the unit meetings. Each unit elects one member to the Board of Directors. Thus, agency policy making is closely tied to front-line needs of foster parents. Foster parents feel that they are supported and involved organizationally as well as from social workers and fellow unit members. Foster parents understand the decisions are made by the board since they select and regularly see their board representatives.

PROFESSIONAL EXPECTATIONS

All members of the PATH team are expected to act in a professional manner. This entails recognizing foster parenting as a legitimate vocational calling requiring education and shared values. Professionalism also includes an expectation that foster parents understand the roles of other professionals and respect the experience, education, and personal involvement of all team members.

Part of being a professional is being paid for services. PATH parents are reimbursed at a rate significantly higher than regular foster parents. The rate is based on days of care and it does not vary according to difficulty. The same rate applies for all foster parents in all areas of the state.

In conclusion, PATH provides an example of how foster parents organize the delivery of foster care services when they are in charge. PATH has built a successful program providing foster family-based treatment to children with a foster parent board and employed professional staff. The key to PATH's success is in developing an organizational environment in which foster parents are supported. This support is found in professional recognition and assistance, clear responsibilities and goals, educational opportunities, administrative services, social work relationships, and unit friendships. The beneficiary of the services is the individual child who is able to receive care in a foster family.

Chapter 17

The Community as an Advocate for Youth: The Programs and Services of the National Youth Advocate Program, Inc.

P. Christopher Kelley
James B. Carruth

ABSTRACT. State treatment foster care programs established by the National Youth Advocate Program are described in terms of youth served, homes established, treatment program, implementation problems, and evaluation procedures.

INTRODUCTION

The National Youth Advocate Program, Inc. (NYAP) was incorporated in Ohio in 1983 as a private, nonprofit youth advocacy organization designed to supervise, guide and develop community-based services for troubled and needy youth. This has been accomplished through various statewide, NYAP-affiliated programs which operate in several states throughout the country and which are responsible for the provision of direct youth advocate programs and services. The National Youth Advocate Program is also actively involved in promoting and developing NYAP subsidiaries in

P. Christopher Kelley is Director of Planning & Program Development at the National Youth Advocate Program, Inc., 1460 West Lane Avenue, Columbus, OH 43221. James B. Carruth is Executive Director of the Ohio Youth Advocate Program, Inc., 145 High Street–Suite 700, Columbus, OH 43215.

other states where there is found to be a definite need for youth advocate program services within those states. The National program provides technical assistance and support services to the state programs, and conducts legal and systems advocacy activities on national and state issues concerning children and youth.

The National Youth Advocate Program, Inc. was actually an outgrowth of its largest state program subsidiary, the Ohio Youth Advocate Program, Inc. (OYAP). OYAP was established in early 1978 as an alternative to institutionalization for youth involved in the juvenile justice, children's services, mental health, and mental retardation systems in Ohio. In 1983, the West Virginia Youth Advocate Program, Inc. was started to serve youth in the northern panhandle of West Virginia. Plans are currently underway to develop a youth advocate program in the state of Indiana.

Since its inception in early 1978, the Ohio Youth Advocate Program has served over 2400 youth. The average current daily census of youth in the Ohio program is between 80 and 85 youth. OYAP currently has 51 licensed foster homes. Since 1983, the West Virginia program has served 159 youth. The average current daily census of youth in the West Virginia program is between 20 and 25 youth, with 20 foster families currently licensed by the program. The daily cost for providing foster care services ranges from $30 to $36 per day, and from $60 to $70 per day for intensive special residential advocate services.

Services provided by both the Ohio and West Virginia programs include specialized foster care, supervised apartment living/independent living services to prepare older adolescents for eventual emancipation, special residential advocacy (intensive, professional foster care provider model), specialized adoption services, and family-based home advocacy services (in-home support services for youth and families in crisis).

The National Youth Advocate Program, Inc. and its state programs were originated from a strong belief that youth who are placed in institutional or correctional facilities are often hurt more than they are helped. It was felt that less restrictive community alternatives using the active involvement and commitment of concerned, caring citizens were needed, and that a youth's family and community are the most valuable resources for positive growth and development. The primary thrust of the youth advocate program is to make such alternatives available to youth and achieve permanency for all our youth through family reunification efforts, independence/emancipation, or adoption. Our programs and services incorporate an advocate model, which involves a one-to-one relationship between a young person and an advocate. Youth in need of supportive, positive role models are assigned an advocate on the basis of mutual interests, compatibility, and personality. These relationships help to provide for the growth and development of the youth's individual strengths and abilities.

Staff of the National Youth Advocate Program, Inc. include its president, director of planning and program development, and administrative support personnel. Each state program has a state director who is responsible for the overall management of the program and a Board of Trustees, comprised of selected representatives from the community at large who have a knowledge of and commitment to youth. The assistant director is responsible for the day-to-day supervision of program staff, intake and placement decisions, and agency compliance to licensure standards. Supervisors are responsible for accessing and monitoring treatment plans and programming for youth, and direct supervision of the area coordinators. The state director, assistant director and supervisors require a minimum of a master's degree in social work or a closely related human services field, and considerable experience in direct youth services and supervision. Area coordinators, or case managers, are responsible for developing and implementing the treatment plan for the youth, foster home and advocate recruitment, training and supervision, and community liaison responsibilities. Area coordinators are required to have a minimum of a bachelor's degree in human services and direct child/youth services experience. Special residential advocates, who provide intensive, professional foster parenting services to very difficult-to-place, special needs adolescents, are required to have a minimum of a bachelor's degree in human services and/or at least one year of experience of working directly with older, special needs youth. All foster parents are recruited based on their dedication, commitment, and skills to parent a troubled and needy adolescent, and their ability to meet agency and state foster home regulations and requirements. An advocate—a mature, stable, and responsible adult recruited from the local community—is assigned to work with a program youth in a one-to-one supportive and friendship relationship based upon mutual interests and compatibility.

CHILDREN AND YOUTH

Due to the nature and flexibility of its individualized programs, the Ohio Youth Advocate Program, Inc. provides services for abused, neglected, dependent, unruly, delinquent, emotionally disturbed, behaviorally maladjusted, mildly and moderately retarded or handicapped children and youth. Generally, OYAP works with any youth who can function with support in a community setting. The age range of these youth is birth to 21 years of age with the majority between 14 and 18 years of age. There is a slightly larger percentage of males, approximately 74 percent of the youth are Caucasian, the balance are Black and other minorities.

Before a youth is accepted for services, certain necessary information regarding the youth must be provided OYAP by the referral agency, including a complete and thorough case history, and any and all psychological/psychiatric reports and evaluations, medical history, written verification of a medical and dental examination within 15 days of placement, school transcripts and immunization records, the youth's birth certificate, the most recent individualized education plan (if applicable), and treatment suggestions from the referring agency, the Medicaid card number and initial ODHS Form 1603 (Review of Child Under Custody). Additional information for a youth to be placed in the temporary custody of OYAP include four certified copies of the juvenile court journal entry awarding custody to OYAP.

With the exception of intake/emergency foster care, all OYAP programs involve an average length of stay of approximately six to 12 months. The long-term goal for each youth in the Ohio Youth Advocate Program is to function in the community in a stable environment. This may include arrangements for an independent living situation, reunifying the youth with the natural family, or another alternative permanent placement. OYAP staff will recommend to the referring agency termination of services for the youth when the goals of his or her personal progress plan have been achieved, and when a satisfactory and more permanent placement has been determined.

The agency has pregnant teens and teen-age mothers in the program. In most cases the referring agency maintains temporary custody of the mother and her infant and allows the infant to be placed in the same foster home as the mother. The agency recruited homes that will accept these teenage mothers and their babies, and find foster parents who are willing to help with teaching child-rearing skills to these young women while, at least in the initial stages of placement, delivering most of the infant care themselves.

FOSTER HOMES

OYAP currently has 51 foster homes, with 31 of the homes being special residential advocate (SRA) homes. All of the foster homes are licensed or approved by either the Ohio Department of Human Services or the Ohio Department of Youth Services. Area coordinator staff recruit prospective foster parents, provide orientation, and complete home studies. Once the home study is approved by the State Office, a recommendation for licensure or approval is sent to the Ohio Department of Human Services of the Ohio Department of Youth Services and the state agency approves or disapproves the recommendation.

Recruitment, orientation, and ongoing training is done on a regional basis, thereby promoting closeness among foster parents in each region that fosters a support group type relationship for foster parents. In all regional monthly training sessions, foster parents are encouraged to share their experiences and knowledge with each other.

Retention of foster parents is accomplished by several methods. First and foremost is making it clear that our agency considers them as the key members of the overall treatment team. This is emphasized when they are recruited and throughout their involvement with our agency. They are actively involved in all decisions relative to their foster youth's treatment plan. Another major factor that affects retention of foster parents is adequate financial reimbursement. Our agency's combined daily board payment and the difficulty-of-care and SRA daily payment to foster parents are among the highest in the state of Ohio, thereby making it less of a financial burden to be foster parents. Last, but not least, are the intensive support services provided by the agency. Line workers, the area coordinators, have relatively small caseloads of ten youth, thereby ensuring much individualized service for these youth and foster parents. In addition to the Area Coordinators, each foster youth is assigned an advocate who works with him or her and the foster parents. The agency maintains a 24-hour, statewide, toll free WATS emergency answering service that can put the foster parents or foster youth in touch with the area coordinator or a supervisor at any time of the day or night, weekdays as well as weekends. This service is very comforting to foster parents since many problems occur at times other than regular business hours.

THE TREATMENT PROGRAM

The area coordinator is responsible for developing the initial treatment plan, the personal progress plan (PPP), with the foster youth, the foster parents, the advocate, and a representative of the referring agency within the first three weeks of placement. This treatment plan is revised as needed and is reviewed at least every six months. The PPP is goal-oriented and includes the following areas: (1) permanency plan; (2) school/education; (3) employment; (4) social services; (5) community involvement; (6) personal growth and development; (7) behavior adjustment; and (8) physical health. In each of these areas the specific tasks, dates the tasks are to be done, and persons responsible for the tasks are noted. Once the plan is final, all parties involved sign the plan, thereby insuring that everyone agrees to the overall goals and that everyone knows his or her tasks and the projected achievement date for those tasks.

The Area Coordinator meets with the youth at least once a week for the first three months of placement and thereafter every two weeks in order to review and evaluate the progress of the youth and the Personal Progress Plan. Depending upon the specific OYAP program, each youth is assigned an advocate (treatment advocate or advocate volunteer) by the area coordinator. The advocate spends 5 hours per week engaged in activities with and on behalf of the youth to assist the youth in achieving the goals of the personal progress plan. At least three-fourths of the required advocate service hours are spent directly with the youth in activities related to the achievement of treatment goals. The balance of the hours may be spent in consultation with the OYAP staff, foster parents, employment, educational, or community resources on behalf of the youth.

The treatment plans always stress the importance of a team approach. All parties involved make a commitment to accomplish specific tasks. Obviously, the greatest commitment of time and energy is that of the foster parents. This is why the foster parents are considered the key members of the treatment team. It is the agency's goal to utilize agency resources and community resources to provide the foster parents with whatever support services are necessary to help them help their foster youth.

The goal of providing support for the foster parents begins with a standardized orientation and preservice training program that the agency provides prior to foster parents having a youth placed in their home. This orientation/preservice training is done on a regional basis in small groups of ten or less; a total of 15 hours of training is accomplished in several sessions held in the evenings or weekends. After the foster parents are licensed they must complete a minimum of 24 hours of inservice training per year (The Ohio Department of Human Services requirement has set a minimum of eight hours of inservice training per year). Foster parents are also encouraged to attend any additional training that relates to foster care. The primary responsibility of the foster parent is to provide a stable family structure in a supportive, supervised living situation which assists the young person in establishing positive relationships within the household and community.

The special residential advocate (SRA) foster parent provides foster care services for youth needing much closer supervision and more intensive services. This program is designed to provide intensive behavior stabilization services for particularly difficult youths, assisting each youth in creating and executing special needs programming, and in obtaining social services and employment and/or educational opportunities with the help of the advocate assigned to the youth. Extensive training and support from agency staff is provided to the SRA as he or she works with very difficult-to-place youths. All SRA's are required to have had previous direct experience and training in working with special needs youth.

The SRA or professional foster parent provides specialized, intensive supervision and support to youth having serious behavioral or emotional problems. In addition, a part-time salaried treatment advocate is assigned to work with the SRA youth on a one-to-one basis. It is one of the agency's goals to accept responsibility and to support policies and practices which protect the community while also assuring justice, concern, and advocacy for youth. Most serious juvenile offenders, behaviorally maladjusted, and mentally handicapped youth who are released from institutional care are eventually returned to their communities. Special residential advocates have the experience and background to work with these youth.

IMPLEMENTATION PROBLEMS

The agency experienced some major problems when the program began in early 1978. Some county Children Services Boards and juvenile courts felt threatened that the agency would recruit established foster parents and that youth with severe social and emotional problems would enter their counties and use limited resources to the detriment of the youth these agencies already had in placement. In some cases, the agency failed to sufficiently explain the program satisfactorily to community leaders and law enforcement agencies as well as local school districts.

A continuing problem has been the recruitment and retention of quality foster parents who are willing to deal with older, more difficult-to-place youth. These foster parents burn out after a period of time and need to take a respite from the rigors of foster parenting.

As with most social service agencies, the recruitment and retention of quality staff is also a problem. After being employed in the social service field for a few years, the reward of helping others with their problems is not sufficient and workers look to positions which offer more financial rewards and more regular employment hours. Our agency is working toward retention of quality personnel by offering health insurance benefits, a retirement plan, and financial bonuses for recruiting and maintaining very difficult and/or minority placements. The agency is also studying the possibility of employment assistants to help the area coordinators with routine paperwork duties and recruitment assistance in order to free up area coordinators' time to concentrate more fully on the treatment aspects of the position.

One of the most significant problems the agency has experienced in implementing and continuing services for youth has been the lack of community resources and involvement for older youths. Many of the youth referred to the agency come from a long history of institutionalization or with extremely poor social skills, school skills, and skills for everyday living. Communities are often not willing to support (either financially or emotionally) a 17-year-old who is only in the tenth grade of school. This youth may have the desire and ability to finish high school, learn a trade, and become a functioning member of society, but very few agencies are willing to underwrite the costs incurred while this youth prepares for eventual emancipation.

The agency tries to work with these youth, assisting them to enroll in trade or vocational schools, encouraging the development of independent living skills, and putting them in contact with public agencies to fill the gap between custodial care and independent living. It is sometimes necessary for the older youth to apply for general relief while attempting to emancipate into the community as a contributing adult.

RESEARCH AND EVALUATION

The majority of youths served during the agency's initial stages of development were referred for foster care from the Ohio Department of Youth Services institutions. This period of foster care was meant to be an interim placement between institutions and return to the youth's home. These youth stayed an average of approximately 6 months before being released.

Since its initial inception in early 1978, OYAP has served approximately 2,400 youth in Ohio; 74 percent of those youth were White, while the remainder were Black and other minorities; 58 percent were males and 42 percent females. The average age of youth entering the program has been 14.5 years.

Success rate of released youths is difficult to determine. When a youth AWOL's from the program, he or she is released unsatisfactorily after a 3-day period. This youth may re-enter the program and ultimately be released satisfactorily. Some referring agencies remove their youths for a variety of reasons before the youth has had a chance to complete the goals of his or her personal progress plan (the major criteria by which successful release versus unsuccessful release is measured). The reasons for these removals are many — lack of funds for foster care placement, agency's desire to have the youth placed closer to his or her home, and so forth. Youths are considered satisfactorily released from the program when the goals of the personal progress plan have been achieved and the youth has not been released to a more restrictive environment. Sixty-one percent of all the youth served by the youth advocate program have achieved successful release.

Length of stay for youth has become progressively longer as the youth enter the program with more severe problems; referring agencies are becoming more willing to let youth who are stable finish out the school year or their high school careers in placement. Currently, the average length of stay is nine months.

During 1983 and 1984 an evaluation was completed of the effectiveness of Youth Advocate Program services as a treatment approach for juvenile delinquents (Selby, 1985). The study compared the treatment effectiveness of the Youth Advocate Program with a large residential treatment center in southwestern Ohio. The major findings of this evaluation study indicate that the Youth Advocate Program does provide significantly more advocacy services and social bonding to youth than the residential treatment center control group. Furthermore, the Youth Advocate Program treatment approach "does have substantial benefit for many problem youths" and has had a substantial measure of success providing services "based upon family treatment at a cost savings to society." While the findings indicated that the use of youth advocates had no substantial influence on determining the outcome of youth behavior, the foster family component had the most positive impact.

The research also showed that the Youth Advocate Program had considerably more success with more problematic youths, primarily as a result of the use of special residential advocate (SRA) foster parents who are required to have more experience and competence than foster care families. "This is another indication of the importance of quality foster homes in determining YAP's program effectiveness." Finally, the research reviewed the kind of values, qualities, and backgrounds which made for the most effective, successful foster families of problem youth within the Youth Advocate Program. As the findings indicated:

> High quality foster families were those with a strong sense of "missionary zeal" expressed towards the cultivation of family life. The most successful foster families appeared to be extremely dedicated to family and to family activity, and to exclude virtually all other interests. Contact with these families revealed that they had comparatively few material possessions and no discernible interest in material acquisition. The prime motivating force for those families was the spiritual value of service to family, friend and neighbor, which was experienced as a joy and pleasure rather than an obligation. Successful foster parents were individuals sustained by nurturing positive growth in others, helping those around them feel good about themselves, and by a steadfast belief that there is no such thing as a bad child. They invariably had a broad extended family network, were very close knit, spent an enormous amount of time on family activities, and considered the foster child to be a full-fledged member of the family.

CONCLUSION

Historically, the Ohio Youth Advocate Program's strength has been its ability to be flexible and responsive to the special needs of foster youth. The agency has served a large number of difficult-to-place foster youth throughout many geographical areas of the state and has been able to maintain a significant rate of success in helping youth and positively impacting on their lives.

There are several identified weaknesses in the program which should be highlighted. Three years ago a decision was made to implement a volunteer advocate model as an experimental project. As such, advocates who were assigned to youth in the foster care program were not paid but were recruited, trained, and assigned to work with foster youth in a volunteer capacity. The volunteer advocate model has not been as effective as the paid advocate model (used for those youths in the SRA program) in providing regular, consistent, ongoing advocate support services to youths. A paid advocate model is more successful in helping to recruit and maintain advocates for youth with more serious presenting problems and needs. The agency was able to attract volunteers to serve as advocates for youth but it was very difficult to retain these volunteer advocates for any substantial period of time. All advocates in the program are now paid, part-time staff members.

A second problem is that regional field offices are maintained and managed by one area coordinator. Any turnover in area coordinator in those offices presents a major disruption of continuity of service to youths, foster parents, and advocates in those areas. An assistant area coordinator position in each regional field office would provide an opportunity to familiarize the assistant area coordinator with the duties and responsibilities of the area coordinator. This would minimize the degree of disruption in maintaining continuity of services and staffing when area coordinator turnover occurs.

A third problem concerns the substantially high number of referrals for older youth (including teenage mothers and their infants) over the past several years. Many of these youth are not able to be reunified with their biological parents. As a result, the agency is experiencing a dramatic need to provide expanded independent living and emancipation services for youth as a viable permanency alternative to family reunification. The agency currently provides some supervised independent and apartment living services for older youth preparing for eventual emancipation; these services need to be developed throughout all areas of the state. We are currently providing additional training for staff and foster parents to assist these youth in independent living transition skills. We are also going to be targeting expanded recruitment and use of independent living residential advocates throughout the state to serve as a viable, transitional program service from foster care to emancipation of older youths.

Chapter 18

Providing Competence Building and Normalizing Environments: The Specialist Family Placement Program of Human Service Associates

Joe Hudson
Burt Galaway
Patricia Harmon

ABSTRACT. Key elements of the HSA service program include contracting, networking, mobilization of community resources, foster parent support systems, and respite care. Procedures for recruiting, licensing, and retaining foster homes are described and implementation difficulties identified.

Human Service Associates is a private agency established in 1979 to provide and promote social services as alternatives to total institutional settings. The agency was organized and developed with a philosophy of least restrictive alternatives and grounded in the notion of normalization to provide structured oportunities within a family setting for youth to develop competencies and accomplish developmental tasks. HSA has evolved over the past eight years,

Joe Hudson is Professor on the Faculty of Social Welfare at the University of Calgary (Edmonton Division), 8625-112th Street, #300, Edmonton, Alberta T6G 1K8 Canada. Burt Galaway is Professor at the School of Social Work, University of Minnesota, 224 Church Street, S.E., #400, Minneapolis, MN 55455. Patricia Harmon is Director of Human Service Associates, Inc., 333 Sibley Street, #111, St. Paul, MN 55101.

expanding from three families and one social worker in 1980, to 90 families and 12 social workers currently providing services to 130 children and youth in the state of Minnesota. The number of service contracts with Minnesota counties has grown from one in 1980 to 37 currently in place. The agency has also expanded the type of services provided, as well as the geographical areas served. In 1983, a respite program component was added, in 1984 services began to be delivered in the state of Wisconsin, and in 1987 specialized foster care services began to be delivered in a rural area of South Carolina. Youth are referred to the HSA program by the child welfare, protection services, and juvenile justice departments of county and state governments.

THE SERVICE PROGRAM

The HSA service program is designed to provide supportive, stable family environments in which young people can accomplish developmental tasks and use community services. The program is organized around five key concepts—contracting, networking, mobilizing community resources, offering a support system, and respite for service providers.

Contracting

All members of the service team are involved in developing written placement agreements to ensure clarity and agreement about reciprocal rights and responsibilities. These agreements and plans identify the specific problems to be addressed, the anticipated length of the placement, the immediate goals or tasks to be accomplished by participants over each three-month period, detailed plans for education, religious participation, medical services, birth family involvement and any special services required by the youth in placement. The preparation of written placement agreements and their monitoring and revision is intended to provide accountability, promote teamwork, and reduce indecision or ambiguity on the part of members of the placement team. Plans evolve over the course of a series of meetings between youth, birth parents, HSA foster parents and social worker, referring agency social worker, as well as other pertinent parties such as special education counselors, or teachers and therapists. Each member of the placement team signs and receives a copy of the placement plan which is then scheduled for review and revised every three months. HSA social workers are responsible for working out the schedule of planning meetings and writing up completed agreements.

Networking

Both birth and foster parents are key persons in the youth's life. The networking efforts of the HSA social worker are aimed at assisting these families in working together to provide a safe, nurturing environment in which the youth can grow through accomplishing developmental tasks. Birth parents, foster parents, and the youth are expected to maintain the nature and type of contact negotiated in the placement plan. The primary social worker for the birth parents is the referring worker who, along with the HSA worker, is expected to facilitate contact and communication between birth parents and youth and assist in resolving any problems. This social network of involved parties to the placement plan amounts to operationalizing the concept of joint parenting by assisting both sets of parents to work cooperatively from their respective strengths in providing care for the youth. This extended family approach is aimed at preventing the fragmentation and detachment that all too often occurs when youth are placed in care. Both foster parents and birth parents are expected to openly communicate and cooperatively work at easing the youth's anxiety about the attachment felt toward both sets of parents. The aim is to encourage the maintenance of links between children in care and their birth parents regardless of whether family reunification is the eventual goal.

Mobilizing Community Resources

Specialized counseling, therapy or other services required for the youth are identified in the placement plan and, in cooperation with the referring agency, arrangements made for their provision. The aim of Human Service Associates is to link youth with existing community resources. This approach was selected for two reasons.

One is the costly potential of HSA duplicating services already available in the community. The other is the normalizing potential of receiving services from a community agency providing services to a variety of other persons from the community rather than having the services provided by the foster care agency only for the youth served. In addition youth will learn how to use community agencies, just as they learn how to use doctors and dentists, and therefore will know where to turn if they require services after leaving foster family care.

Foster Parent Support System

Foster parenting is a difficult and emotionally draining activity frequently made more difficult by a sense of isolation and lack of support. To help in this, HSA requires that agency foster parents participate in monthly support group meetings. The group purpose is one of providing mutual support from which foster parents can derive strength, encouragement, and access to a web of supportive relationships with others dealing with similar problems, tasks, and responsibilities. Foster parents are organized into groups of no more than ten that meet in a convenient location. The HSA social worker who works with the group members also attends, but foster parents are expected to take the lead in directing and structuring the work of the group. The HSA social worker is responsible for facilitating and assisting, not directing or leading group meetings. Each support group is eligible to receive $200 each year from the agency to assist in covering programming costs. These funds are available for each unit, according to the specific programming costs the unit determines are needed; the only requirement is that each unit submit a report at the end of the year on how the funds were used. Support groups are not intended to meet training requirements but, instead, achieve mutual aid, problem solving, emotional support and teamwork building of group members. In addition, each licensed foster parent receives a $200.00 per year training allowance with which to select applicable training or educational experiences. Finally, HSA provides training opportunities for foster parents through workshops presented by the agency.

Respite Care

Respite is a period of rest or relief available to agency foster parents and designed to provide a temporary break from the daily challenges of caring for a foster child. The HSA respite program is designed to provide a safe, nurturing environment for youth while providing a respite resource for the foster care givers. All agency foster parents are provided with compensated accrued time off at the rate of one-half day for each calendar month the year is in placement, up to a maximum of 6 days during a calendar year. In turn, each respite provider is licensed as a foster parent by HSA and expected to meet agency service standards. Written respite agreements are prepared covering the anticipated respite schedule, transportation arrangements, responsibilities of each party and specific plans for the respite stay. Whenever possible, pre-respite visits are arranged prior to the actual stay. Foster parents who act as respite providers are organized into support group units, in the same way as other foster parents in the agency, are regarded as full members of the agency service team, and expected to be involved in all decisions concerning the respite services provided.

FOSTER HOME RECRUITMENT, LICENSURE, AND RETENTION

HSA foster parents range in age from 21 to 67, are married or single, and live in both rural and metropolitan areas of each state. Foster parents are recruited and licensed through a group orientation and training process and are sought from a variety of ethnic and socioeconomic backgrounds. Experienced foster parents and those with professional or life experiences compatible with the skills needed in fostering are selected.

HSA uses a variety of ongoing recruitment means. Close contact is maintained with state foster parent organizations in which HSA foster parents are encouraged to actively participate. The agency covers all costs associated with foster parents attending annual state conferences and has taken the initiative at organizing conference sessions and sponsoring social hours and information booths. More traditional types of advertising are also used, including advertisements in community newspapers, posters, brochures and radio advertising. A speaker's bureau is maintained by the agency and foster parents and social workers are encouraged to speak to local groups who have indicated an interest in learning more about the work of the agency. Emphasis is placed on recruiting foster parents from populations of color and currently over one-third of agency parents are persons of color. Orientation and pre-service training for prospective foster parents takes place in a series of group meetings designed to provide information about the agency, the nature of the work undertaken, and necessary skills. The aim is to provide prospective care givers with sufficient information to make reasoned choices about foster parenting with HSA. A standard format is used in orientation meetings to define service team roles and expectations and provide a positive and realistic image of foster parenting. Prospective foster parents are encouraged to discuss their motivations openly and ask questions freely. Topical areas covered in orientation sessions include the following:

- A description of the agency, its philosophy and history
- Relevant legal information, including Public Law 96-272 and the American Indian Child Welfare Act
- The nature of the agency team concept and the roles of team members
- Expectations of agency foster parents, including participation in support groups, training, respite and social worker/foster parent working relationships
- Expectation of including birth parents as part of the team
- Information on the placement and licensing processes
- Description of the characteristics of youth placed

Currently licensed HSA foster parents are encouraged to attend and play an active role in the orientation sessions.

Extensive information is collected from prospective foster parents and compiled in the form of a pre-licensing home study. Included is information on the reasons for wanting to become a foster family, the developmental history of the family, and its current functioning. Particular attention is given to the capacity of the marriage to withstand a foster child, the role each parent plays in the family, and the nature of interaction and division of labor between family members. Particular attention is given to community and extended family support systems for licensed single parents. Key questions assessed in the licensing study concern the extent to which the family will allow a foster child to enter and become an integral part of the family and the foster family's ability to work as an extension of the natural family. The HSA social worker is responsible for licensing foster parents and conducting annual performance evaluations at the time of re-licensure. Each licensed foster parent is expected to complete a minimum of 18 hours formal training each year, defined broadly to include educational classes, workshops, seminars, and conferences.

The age of the youth placed by HSA range from a few days to 19. For youths two and above, the primary reasons for placement are abuse and neglect, emotional disturbances, and delinquency. A smaller number of this group are mentally retarded and physically handicapped youth. Usually the youth aged two and younger are being referred to HSA for placement in a black or Indian home because birth parents are unable to care for them and homes of color are less readily available in the county foster care systems.

Retaining qualified foster parents is as important as recruitment and licensure. HSA has experienced little foster parent turnover largely as a result of providing prospective foster parents with accurate information about the agency and the expectations held for them, providing foster parents with full opportunities to participate in decision-making about placement and programming, and providing ongoing training and support to help decrease the probability of foster parent burnout.

EVALUATION RESEARCH

Human Service Associates recently implemented a two-track evaluation system, composed of an ongoing monitoring system and periodic program evaluation studies. The ongoing monitoring system is aimed at supplementing administrative records and building on data currently being collected. The system is designed to provide monthly, quarterly, and annual reports from data in four files. The first file deals with foster home inquiries and provides information on the initial inquiry up to a licensing decision. The second file covers homes licensed up to the time of termination. The third file covers youth referral information up to the placement decision, and the fourth file contains placement information up to the time of termination, including a three- and six-month follow-up on all youth served.

The second part of the agency evaluation system involves planning and conducting periodic studies on specific program elements. Periodic evaluation studies are designed to supplement the ongoing information system and provide more detailed information on specific program questions. The primary clients for these studies are program managers, including social service supervisors and state directors. The aim is to conduct a minimum of three evaluation studies of key agency service components during the course of any year and to involve agency social workers and foster parents as active participants in the study design and implementation.

A recently completed study dealt with placement planning and service agreements. Methods used involved drawing a sample of completed service agreements and assessing them against criteria derived largely from agency policies having to do with the timeliness, consistency, and completeness of the information reported. Particular attention was given to persons participating, planning for the youth's permanent living situation, the nature and number of quarterly goals established and assessed for each party to the service agreement, and the expected type and amount of involvement by the birth parents and other family members. Information reported from this study is being used in supervisory and training sessions with agency foster parents and social workers. HSA social workers and foster parents were involved in the data collection phase of the study and will have a sense of ownership in the results and a commitment to improving the quality of services provided. The ideal sought is that of a self-evaluating organization, constantly monitoring operations and collecting, assessing and using information for program improvement.

IMPLEMENTATION

Major implementation difficulties associated with the HSA specialized foster care program amounted to using an entrepreneurial vehicle to deliver a relatively new type of service with no start-up capital for which key referral agents had little information. These difficulties interacted and compounded each other and continue to exist today, although in modified form.

HSA was incorporated and implemented by three social workers, each holding separate full-time positions and none with substantial amounts of money. The agency literally began with some stationery, a telephone number and telephone located in the office of another social agency whose director was willing to have staff answer and take HSA messages. The lack of funds meant that there were no full-time employees in the agency and the incorporators had to take vacation time from their regular employment in order to carry out necessary implementation activities. Hiring full-time social work staff was beyond the financial abilities of the agency and therefore a deliberate policy decision was taken to pay social workers on the same basis as the special services foster parents to be recruited. Just as foster parents would be paid on the basis of the number of days of service provided to children placed, so social workers would be paid on the number of children placed in homes recruited and licensed by them. With no children placed, social workers would not be paid. This system amounted to sharing financial risk between all significant parties in the agency—the Board of Directors, social workers, and foster parents. While necessary, the policy was seen as rather unorthodox and unattractive to many social workers who would otherwise have been interested in employment with the agency.

The policy of paying on a per diem basis shaped and targeted the recruitment of social workers toward those persons able and willing to assume some degree of financial risk, at least to the extent that it was outweighed by a desire to build a specialist fostering caseload within a small, new, and private agency. More dramatically, the payment policy had the effect of slowing the growth of the agency. For example, during the first year, only one social worker joined the agency and during the second, another. In turn, this meant that fewer specialist parents could be recruited and licensed, and referrals could not be accepted from county agencies who may have been interested in using agency services. This problem of slow growth was anticipated by the founders at the time of establishing the agency. The only options available were to borrow substantial amounts of money from a friendly banker or seek a grant from a private foundation. The first option was rejected because none of the incorporators would likely have been seen as a good financial risk, nor would the business venture be seen as having particularly good prospects. The option of securing funding from a private foundation was rejected because of a desire to operate the agency as an entrepreneurial activity, and foundations were not able to fund for-profit business.

The second major implementation difficulty had to do with the decision to incorporate and operate Human Service Associates on a for-profit basis. The notion of an entrepreneurial human services agency was foreign in 1979 and, while perhaps less so today, continues to be viewed in some circles with skepticism and distrust. A host of negative stereotypes tend to be associated with for-profit agencies delivering social services, including notions about making money off human misery and maximizing profits at the expense of service quality. What these ideas fail to consider is that all persons, whether employed in public or private not-for-profit social welfare agencies, generate income from difficulties being experienced by their clients. Fair compensation for services rendered is the key principle that should drive the activities of all people delivering services, regardless of whether the agency employing them is public, private not-for-profit, or private for-profit.

The notion that for-profit agencies aim at maximizing profit and sacrificing service quality is a kind of reflex notion that, under more careful consideration, fails to hold. John Kenneth Galbraith (1967) attempted to dispel this notion but it continues to persist. It simply makes little sense to expect that a business will succeed if attention is not given to delivering quality services. To aim at maximizing profit at the expense of service quality is both amateurish and self-defeating. An agency operating on that basis would likely have a very short life. And deservedly so. A second point to consider in respect to the argument about maximizing profits is that what is labelled profit in a for-profit agency and what is labeled an expense in a not-for-profit agency amounts to an accounting convenience. Public agencies and private nonprofit agencies aim at ensuring that government allocations and expected income equal anticipated expenses. What gets lumped into the expense category, however, can often be seen as indirect types of income or fringe benefits. For example, a nonprofit agency can use additional monies to increase the salaries of staff, enhance travel benefits, and obtain and furnish more elaborate office space. The incentive may not be one of operating efficiently but more one of ensuring that no monies accrue at the end of the fiscal year. The success of the agency then gets measured by the variety of accoutrements provided the service providers.

The foreign nature of a for-profit social services agency and the skepticism and distrust likely to be generated were anticipated by the HSA board members at the time of incorporating and establishing the agency. It was well appreciated that such perceptions might slow the development of the agency. Even in light of such sober assessments a decision was made to proceed with an entrepreneurial agency out of a belief in the free enterprise system and the benefits of enhancing the efficiency of the agency.

The third major implementation problem confronting the development of Human Service Associates had to do with the relative novelty of the services being delivered. County administrators equated the services offered by HSA as essentially the same as the foster care services delivered by their own social services departments. This problem continues to be addressed by providing information to these decision makers about the HSA program and the target group to be served. We emphasize that HSA is not in the business of competing with traditional county foster care programs but very much in the business of competing with residential treatment centers. A crucial element in reaching a better understanding with county administrators is providing them with information about the number of children being referred outside the county to residential treatment centers and the costs incurred for such placements. With that kind of information and fuller appreciation of the HSA service program, many county administrators encourage their social work staff to begin making some referrals to HSA and, based on satisfaction with these initial referrals, increasing numbers have followed.

Chapter 19

The New Brunswick
Therapeutic Home Program

Reuben Orenstein

ABSTRACT. A Canadian province-wide specialist fostering scheme is described in terms of the children served, homes licensed, program services provided, and implementation difficulties.

INTRODUCTION

New Brunswick is a largely rural, small eastern Canadian province with approximately 725,000 people, bounded on the north by the province of Quebec, on the south by the province of Nova Scotia, and to the west by the state of Maine. Approximately 60 percent of its people speak English and 40 percent speak French. Most of the population is Caucasian; only two percent are Indian, Metis, or Black. New Brunswick is classed by the federal government as a have-not province. Nearly ten percent of the adult population is in receipt of social assistance, compared with less than seven percent nationally. The unemployment rate in the province for the month of July, 1987 was 12.5 percent, but only 8.5 percent for Canada as a whole.

Therapeutic home services are provided by the New Brunswick Department of Health and Community Services through its 11 regional offices. Traditionally, the Department has relied heavily on

Reuben Orenstein is Program Consultant at Children's Residential Services, Department of Health and Community Services, Post Office Box 5100, Fredericton, New Brunswick E3B 5G8 Canada.

235

family dwellings to meet the needs of children in care, including children with emotional disabilities. Although group home and institutional setting have been used, the foster home remains the placement of choice for most children. The foster home program, however, has not kept pace in recent years with the changes in the Department's child welfare practices. Since the 1970s, the Department has intervened early and intensively with families to prevent children from coming into care. As a result, children who do come into care tend to be older and have serious emotional problems stemming from traumatic family backgrounds.

The need to find appropriate resources for this growing population of children was borne out in a departmental study carried out in 1979 on the needs of children in care, and again in 1980 on the characteristics of foster and group home resources in the provinces. Key findings from these two studies revealed the following:

- 60 percent of children in care have some degree of behavioral and emotional problems.
- 48 percent of the more disturbed children had between two and ten placement changes within a two-year span, and at the time of the study, 75 percent of this same group were in fairly new or unstable placements.
- 30 percent of the more seriously disturbed children changed their last placement due either to behavior problems or at their own request.
- 75 percent of the foster parents surveyed indicated that they would not accept a child with acting-out problems, such as running away, taking drugs, or stealing.
- 16 percent of the foster homes used by children in the 1979 study were closed one year later.
- 37 percent of the foster parents surveyed said that they were not prepared to accept any new children due mainly to their age and demands of the jobs.

The therapeutic home program first began in 1982 as an alternative to developing a group home in the Campbellton region in the northern part of the province. The second program started in Fredericton, the provincial capital, the following year, and by 1984, a provincial program design was put in place with service standards enacted the year after.

Therapeutic homes are presently operating in six regions and one branch office with plans to expand the program in the remaining five regions as resources become available. As of August, 1987, there were 40 therapeutic homes across the province serving 48 children. Fifty-one therapeutic homes have been approved and have served over 100 children since the program's inception. The cost of providing therapeutic care for a child is $680.64 a month (Canadian). This rate covers basic food, clothing, and personal effects as well as a fee-for-service for the time and skill required to help the child. Therapeutic parents are entitled to four seasonal allowances that cover the cost of extra clothing and recreation supplies in addition to the monthly rate. Special services such as tutoring, counselling, and respite care are also available on an as-needed basis.

DESCRIPTION OF THE CHILDREN SERVED

The child is capable of fitting into a family environment and developing a relationship to some extent. The child has some degree of impulse control. Boys and girls of all ages are served by the program. Over 60 boys and 40 girls have been placed, ranging in age from 7 to 19 years. The majority of children served are 14 years of age and over. An agreement of order is required to rationalize the Department's intervention with the child and to ensure that terms of a service agreement with the natural family are carried out. In addition to behavior problems, physical, mental and learning disabilities may also be present. The child must not be bedridden or require total nursing care. Some extreme behavior problems are not acceptable, including demonstrated irrational violence toward persons and compulsive fire setting.

All of the children placed are referred by the Department of Health and Community Services. Most of the children are in care; a few are young offenders. The worker for the child makes the referral to the therapeutic home coordinator, who, in turn, discusses the child with the therapeutic parents at their next group session. Involving the therapeutic parents in the referral process ensures commitment to the child once placed in a therapeutic home.

THE THERAPEUTIC HOME

A therapeutic home is a foster home approved to accept and work with one or two children who are emotionally disturbed and may have other disabilities; the foster parents will also work with the child's natural family, if appropriate. The best source of therapeutic homes is among the Department's existing foster families. Foster families have often been doing the job of therapeutic parents, often without the recognition, support, or financial remuneration they deserve. A recruitment campaign may be launched only after all appropriate foster parents have been approved and there still remains a need for more homes.

The following criteria are considered in recruiting potential therapeutic homes:

1. The therapeutic family should possess characteristics of a close-knit healthy family.

   a. A therapeutic parent should have the same qualities that are expected from any good foster parent. These include non-possessive warmth, empathic understanding, patience, self-confidence, humility, consistency, and a sense of humor.

   b. The therapeutic family should demonstrate healthy dynamics and elicit good interpersonal relationships among all family members.

   c. Family member roles should be clearly defined and accepted by all.

   d. There should be evidence of good marital, parent-child and sibling communications, with a healthy respect of all members for each other.

2. All family members, including the children of the therapeutic parents, must accept and participate, to the extent of their abilities, in the program.

3. The therapeutic family's religious, social, and cultural value system should be reasonably compatible with the child's background and treatment needs.

4. The therapeutic parents should be prepared to work in a mutual support system with other therapeutic parents.

5. Therapeutic parents should be prepared to work closely with professionals, as team members.

6. Therapeutic parents should possess basic knowledge of how children grow and develop. In addition, they should be willing and able to participate in training sessions in order to conceptualize innate skills and learn new ones.

7. Therapeutic parents should be able to contribute to and follow a treatment plan.

8. Therapeutic parents should be prepared to accept and work with the child's natural parents. They should be understanding and tolerant of a wide range of dysfunctional behavior, such as alcoholism, abuse, and incest. They should welcome natural parents into their home, as arranged, and, through a helping relationship, model more effective communication and parenting skills. They should be prepared to share parenting responsibilities with natural parents, such as maintaining contact with their child's school.

9. The motivation to become a therapeutic home should be based on the reality that therapeutic parents experience disappointments, frustrations, and failure as well as success.

10. The therapeutic family should have community roots and/or be prepared to reside where they are for some time.

THE THERAPEUTIC PROGRAM

The primary purpose of a therapeutic home is to provide time-limited care and treatment of an emotionally disturbed child who is expected to improve to the extent that he or she can successfully be placed home with his or her natural family, or in a less demanding environment such as a foster home or an independent living environment. Length of placement varies with each child, but the expected period is between six months and two years.

Occasionally, the therapeutic family and their child whose permanency plan is long-term foster care will develop a strong mutual bond. In such a case, the therapeutic parents may request that the child remain in their home on an indefinite basis. If this is acceptable to all parties, the status of the home as a treatment resource for this child or others may be reexamined. If the child has made significant gains in his or her behavior and general deportment to the point where he or she no longer needs the therapeutic program, the home may then be reassessed as a regular foster home, with a resulting reduction in financial benefits and service input from the worker. Therapeutic homes are usually approved for one child only. In a limited number of cases, a second child may be placed, if the worker and therapeutic parents concur, but only after the first child has settled and some of the presenting problems have subsided.

Attendance and participation in peer group supervision is the major service support received by the therapeutic parents. The group functions as a simulated extended family, a single, interacting, interdependent system. Although each therapeutic family has primary responsibility for the child placed in their home, they also have a secondary responsibility for the children placed with other couples in the same extended family group. Four of five therapeutic families in a region constitute a group. Each group is facilitated by the therapeutic home worker in the region. The groups meet regularly on a biweekly basis for two to three hours and serve several functions — education, treatment planning, and support. Didactic information is provided by the worker and other clinically-oriented professionals who also help provide new insights for therapeutic parents to deal more effectively with disturbed behavior. Functioning as a team, the therapeutic parents and social worker define the child's problems, establish treatment goals, devise strategies to achieve these goals, and review results. No particular treatment intervention is advocated or promoted by the Department. Instead, the values and skills of each individual therapeutic family is employed and enhanced to meet the needs of the child who is selected for placement. The group must become cohesive. Therapeutic parents are encouraged to openly express their thoughts and feelings (both positive and negative), share experiences, provide emotional support, and help out with practical advice.

The success of the therapeutic home program depends heavily on the availability and involvement of the assigned staff member. A full-time worker assigned to the program is preferred. Where this is not feasible due to resource restrictions and/or fewer families and children, an appropriate reduction in the size of the worker's regular caseload is made to reflect the additional input these children and therapeutic families require. The therapeutic home worker carries out several functions including:

1. Recruiting and assessing therapeutic home applicants (in conjunction with the foster home coordinator).
2. Providing training to therapeutic families.
3. Facilitating group meetings.
4. Working with natural parents or liaising with the worker for the natural parents about coordination of treatment plans.
5. Visiting the child (at least once a month).
6. Consulting with individual therapeutic families.
7. Liaising with external agencies.
8. Evaluating individual treatment families.

IMPLEMENTATION

Successful programs in Canada, most notably the Parent Counsellors program in Alberta and the Parent Therapist program at the Chedoke-McMaster Centre, Hamilton, Ontario, were examined prior to implementing the program on a province-wide scale. Meetings were held with several parent counselors in Edmonton, Alberta to discuss the program and get a sense of what therapeutic parents were like. We were impressed with the dedication and commitment shown by these parents and with their humaneness and vulnerability. For example, when asked what type of child was *not* acceptable in their homes, after a brief pause, one parent offered that she could not accept a child who was fat! This point struck home, for in the end it is the respect for the unique qualities of each individual family that makes the program work, rather than the uniform application of a selected intervention technique. The practice of approving existing foster families rather than recruiting new ones was *not* practiced either in Ontario or Alberta. It was a good decision for New Brunswick, however, due to the small, tight-knit fostering communities in the province. To overlook those families who were doing the job with everything but title or money would be perceived as an insult and could result in increased attrition. Membership in the program is an incentive for other foster families to strive to achieve.

The program was piloted in one community for six months to test the recruitment, assessment, and group support systems. Following this process, provincial program standards were developed and enforced. A therapeutic home has the potential of replacing the need for a more specialized residential treatment center or institution for many disturbed children. With appropriate training and supervision, a therapeutic parent is able to bring to the job the same relationship-building skills and behavioral change elements as child caring staff in residential centers or institutions. Therapeutic parents provide a unique program tailored to the needs of the child that is often difficult to do in group care settings.

On a practical level, therapeutic homes are much easier to set up and operate than residential centers. Per diem costs are considerably lower. Therapeutic homes, however, do not totally replace the need for residential centers for all children. Some very aggressive children require a degree of security that can only be guaranteed in more complex facilities. Some extremely deprived children also require so much time and effort from care givers that only in settings where staff share the children by working shifts can these children be effectively treated.

CONCLUSIONS

During the five years that the therapeutic home program has been operating in New Brunswick a number of strengths have been noted:

1. A therapeutic home placement is a less detrimental alternative for an emotionally disturbed child compared with a treatment center or institution, and conforms with the principle of normalization.
2. Therapeutic home placements provide highly individualized treatment.
3. Therapeutic homes are relatively easy to set up and administer. In New Brunswick, therapeutic homes are paid and maintained through the department's general child welfare maintenance system.

4. The program is flexible and readily adaptable to meet regional needs.

Among its weaknesses:

1. Therapeutic homes are subject to the same supply-and-demand pressures as the regular foster home system. The more successful a therapeutic home program is in a region, the more there are demands on its services.
2. Some attrition is a reality, despite efforts at development and retention. Since therapeutic parenting is not a career or a salaried position, the decision by therapeutic parents to continue is based on the personal needs of individual family members.

Therapeutic homes are expected to expand to all regions by the end of the decade. Due to their relative scarcity, therapeutic homes are perceived as regional resources only. Once the number of homes expand, they will become part of a provincial network of placement options.

Chapter 20

The Hampshire (England) Adult Placement Scheme

Leigh A. Jones

ABSTRACT. An innovative specialist fostering scheme established in Hampshire, England is described with particular attention given to clients served, benefits of adult placements and problem areas needing attention.

INTRODUCTION

Hampshire, situated in Central Southern England, is one of the largest counties in Britain with a population of approximately one and a half million. It is the main center of population on the south coast belt, which includes Southampton and Portsmouth, and in the north of the county at Basingstoke and Aldershot. Between these urban areas, there is a large area of countryside, interspersed with market towns and small villages. The standard of living is high, but here are areas of severe urban deprivation.

The Hampshire Adult Placement Scheme was established by Hampshire County Council's Social Services Department in 1979. The original aim was to place people with mental handicap or mental illness with approved families, known as carers, although it was always intended that the scheme would expand to include elderly people and people with a physical handicap. This expansion oc-

Leigh A. Jones is affiliated with the Social Service Department at Fareham Health Centre, Civic Way, Osborn Road, Fareham, Hants PO16 7ED United Kingdom.

245

curred in 1981, when the number of adult placement officers was increased from three to six. A short-stay scheme was also established at this time, and in 1982 each of the 17 Social Services Area Centers recruited an adult placement social worker to identify suitable clients for placement and offer support to those clients and their families before and during placement. The role of the adult placement officer was to recruit and support carers and have prime responsibility for matching carer and client.

The maximum number of clients placed per household is three. The scheme has grown from 48 carers able to accommodate 102 clients as of January 1, 1980, to 267 carers able to accommodate 494 clients as of January 1, 1987. From 1979 through 1986 the scheme had 2,026 applications for long-stay placements and placed 72 percent (1,458) of the applicants. Thirteen percent (183) of the placements were elderly, 64 percent (936) were mentally handicapped, 17 percent (344) mentally ill, and six percent (85) were persons with physical handicaps. Six hundred and sixty-five short-stay placements were made, of which 30 percent (199) were elderly, 56 percent (372) were mentally handicapped, six percent (40) were mentally ill, and eight percent (35) were persons with physical handicaps. The placement of people with mental handicaps continues to be the main focus of the scheme, although further expansion of the scheme in 1988 will emphasize placement of physically handicapped and elderly people.

The Adult Placement Scheme has the following aims:

a. To widen the range of choice of accommodation for adults who require family placement as a result of age, disability, or past or present illness, whether for a specified time or an indefinite period.

b. To assist clients to achieve their aim of living with a caring family in ordinary housing.

c. To enable clients who have lived with a carer for a period of time to move, if they wish, to a more independent setting.

d. To promote a philosophy which emphasizes the individuality, value, and dignity of all people in placement.

e. To recruit carers able to provide clients with a valued lifestyle.

f. To ensure that clients in placement are able to take as full as possible advantage of community facilities.

g. To form part of a comprehensive community care program involving liaison with other service providers.

h. To provide a cost-effective service, but to arrange placements based on client need, not on grounds of cost.

Placement Officer:
- Advertise for and recruit carers
- Support carers
- Match carer and client
- Arrange finances
- Control carer resource

Social Worker:
- Identify clients for placement
- Liaise with placement officer
- Support client before, during, and following placement
- Arrange reviews on each client

Joint Roles:
- Encourage other professionals to "think positively about adult placement
- Public education

POSITIVE ASPECTS OF ADULT PLACEMENT

There is a growing move in Britain towards community care as a more appropriate provision than large institutional settings; in Hampshire the large hospitals for mental handicap and mental illness are planned for closure, except for a very small group of patients who cannot safely be placed in the community.

The scheme also considers people for placement who are living with relatives who are finding it difficult to cope, e.g., elderly people living with relatives, or people with mental handicap being cared for by an elderly parent. The vast majority of elderly people continue to lead an active life in their own homes without the need for assistance. Many others will cope with the benefit of domiciliary and day-care services or will move to sheltered housing. There is, however, a growing minority who require a higher level of care than can be provided in their own homes.

The traditional option has been to offer accommodation in a local authority residential home or in private homes for the elderly. Although some very frail people require such accommodation, placing large groups of elderly people together in a congregate facility is an unsatisfactory option for people who have spent most of their lives as active participants in the community. In considering adult placement as an option, the following positive aspects can be highlighted and are frequently absent from larger institutions:

a. The retention of personal dignity and privacy.
b. The meeting of emotional as well as physical needs.
c. The retention of strong links with the community.
d. Being able to remain in the home area, if requested.

All clients placed under adult placement have their own single bedrooms, with their own possessions, including items of furniture. They will be able to continue to undertake everyday activities, or will be trained to do so if they have never been able to undertake particular tasks, e.g., shopping, gardening, using public transport, ironing, etc. If clients are in need of personal physical care, they will be able to enjoy the dignity of being offered that care at a personal level on a one-to-one basis, rather than by whoever happens to be on duty at the time.

After receiving an application form, the adult placement officer will interview the client with his or her social worker and will attempt to identify a suitable carer vacancy. A suitable vacancy may already be available or advertising for a new carer may be necessary. When clients are unsure whether they wish to live with a family or carer vacancy cannot be identified immediately, a short-story placement may be offered with a carer from the short-stay pool to give the client an opportunity to sample family life.

When a suitable long-term vacancy has been identified, the adult placement officer liaises with the client's social worker, who initiates client introductory visits to the carer. The matching process will then proceed at the individual pace of carer and client; informal contact will hopefully accelerate before the trial placement occurs. A trial placement period of a minimum of four weeks precedes a decision to make the placement long-term.

PROBLEM AREAS

Reluctance of some professionals to fully accept the option of family placement for adults has been one of the main problems. A redirection of professional thinking is required with adult placement introduced as an option before residential care is discussed. A factor in reluctance to consider adult placement may be that the matching process is generally more time-consuming when introducing a client to a carer than to residential care. There are more subtle aspects to take into account, such as matching of personalities between carer and client and between client and other clients already in placement.

Relatives' views and reactions to adult placement need to be carefully considered. There will frequently be feelings of guilt that another family is being asked to cope with their relative when they themselves were unable to cope. It is vital to involve relatives in the introductory process and to allow them the opportunity to initiate informal contact with carers before placement proceeds. The final decision, however, as to whether the placement goes ahead lies with the carer and client.

The availability of suitable accommodation is a problem. Many elderly clients will be unable to climb stairs and while some families are willing to convert a spare downstairs room into a bedroom, the bathroom and toilet are frequently upstairs. The use of commodes in bedrooms is discouraged. Procedures regarding necessary remodeling must be agreed to with the occupational therapy department of the local authority running the placement scheme. In Hampshire there is an agreed policy that priority will be given to essential adaptations in the home of carers and that such work will be undertaken before a client is placed.

Carer recruitment is an important issue for the success of any scheme. Some families organize themselves in a very structured way; it is vital to select carers able to deal flexibly with people's needs and treat them as individuals. For example, carers are encouraged to allow clients to deal with their own medication, even though there may be a small element of risk involved. Carer flexibility can be arranged by training to cover specific topics such as awareness therapy for confused elderly people, management of incontinence, and so forth.

Finally, common sense and realism must guide the assessment of client suitability for adult placement. Not everyone can be successfully placed. We have had difficulty placing clients who have low motivation for living with a family, who have extremely difficult behavior problems or a regular history of physical violence, who are incontinent day and night on a regular basis, who are confused and keep the family awake all night, or who are very frail requiring 24-hour nursing care.

SUPPORT FOR CARER AND CLIENT

Both personal and practical support must be available to carer and client for a successful scheme. Most important is the necessity of continued personal support to carer and client from the adult placement officer and social worker respectively. Separate support ensures that the workers involved will not have conflicting interests; it enables the carer and client to talk freely about any problems, and the social worker providing client personal support gives the scheme organizer more time to develop the scheme's resources.

Support is also provided through careful planning and use of information. Reviews are held every six months and are always held in the carer's home with carer and client present for the whole of the meeting. Prior to placement the client signs an agreement form which includes consent to the passing on of any confidential information to the carer. The assessment of potential carers includes safeguards such as a request for two references, completion of a medical form, and written confirmation of all previous criminal convictions.

Several forms of practical support are provided. Holiday relief is provided for up to three weeks per year for the carer. The client will either go to his or her own family, stay with another carer, or arrange for a holiday during these three weeks. This arrangement is vital for ongoing success of the placement and the carer is actively encouraged to make use of this provision.

Day-care is arranged for the client if appropriate and is not limited to the traditional forms of day-care. Day-care, for example, may be at a leisure or work establishment. Board and lodgings payments to the carer are usually arranged through the Department of Health and Social Security (DASS), although some clients will be able to pay from their own private means. A supplement can be paid for clients in full-time employment if their pay is insufficient to meet the board and lodging charges. The Adult Placement Scheme may assist carers from its own budget with interim refunding loans paid to the carer at the beginning of a placement when there is a delay in receipt of payment from DHSS. The loans may also be used for holiday and short-stay placements, clothing grants, compensation outside normal insurance claims for damages caused by clients, and for furniture such as beds, mattresses, and special chairs.

CONCLUSION

The time has come for family placement of adults to develop into a key provision in a range of services. Mr. Jerome illustrates the potential for family placement of adults:

> Mr. Jerome, aged 49, was first referred to the adult placement scheme via a case review held in January. He had been a resident at a hostel for younger physically disabled people for several years following the diagnosis of a brain tumor. Although recovering well after initial fears of a poor prognosis, Mr. Jerome suffered severe short-term memory loss and needed care in a residential setting. A number of problems were highlighted initially, including Mr. Jerome's lack of motivation toward movement, his financial situation, and the views of his family. In June a newly approved carer was identified as a possibility for a short-term placement for Mr. Jerome; after introductory meetings this plan went ahead. He thoroughly enjoyed the week and on return to the hostel he began packing his bags. Mr. Jerome returned to the carer for a long-term trial period. A case review was held two weeks later which both the client and carer attended. Mr. Jerome has been settled with the carer five years and has settled remarkably well to a busy, friendly, and fairly disorganized family life. He has con-

founded professionals' fears that he would be unable to cope with a change of this magnitude. In fact, he has benefited significantly, enjoying the sense of humor in the household and behaving in a more relaxed and cheerful manner. Day-care is now being arranged at a local occupational therapy center to provide Mr. Jerome with an outside interest and to offer a break for the carer.

A working party should be formed to identify schemes already in operation, identity common practices, issue guidelines for operation and practice standards, and encourage development of additional schemes.

CONCLUSION

Chapter 21

Specialist Fostering:
Themes and Issues

Burt Galaway
Joe Hudson

ABSTRACT. Specialist foster family care has quietly developed in the last twenty years and consistently reflects features of families' services providing within their homes, receiving payment for services, and are the primary service providers with social workers and other staff providing back-up supervision and consultation. Matters for consideration as this programming thrust develops include distinguishing models of service which define the problem as lying with the child who is assumed to require treatment contracted with models which take a more ecological approach, clarifying the roles of foster parents and social workers, specifying the role of birth parents in specialist foster family care programs, developing the relationship of specialist foster family care to permanency planning, and identifying possible future directions including more extensive use of this type of service for adults.

Burt Galaway is Professor at the School of Social Work, University of Minnesota, 224 Church Street S.E., #400, Minneapolis, MN 55455. Joe Hudson is Professor on the Faculty of Social Welfare, University of Calgary (Edmonton Division), 8625-112th Street, #300, Edmonton, Alberta T6G 1K8 Canada.

253

The nineteen papers in this volume present a fascinating glimpse of a new form of community care which has been quietly emerging over the last 20 years. Specialist fostering incorporates the substitute family ingredients of traditional foster family care and the systematic interventions characteristic of residential treatment. The programs involve placing troubled children and youth with families who have been selected, trained, and supervised to cope with the behavior and meet the developmental needs of these children and youth. The different names used to describe the programs—treatment foster care, specialized foster care, specialist family care, professional foster care, family-based treatment, and community care—reflect the different service models and orientations used in the programs and their development under different administrative auspices. The roots of these programs go back to the establishment of difficulty-of-care rates which were made available in the 1960s to foster parents who were prepared to accept and cope with children requiring special care. Several specialist foster family care programs emerged in the early 1970s including the PATH program in Minnesota (Galaway, 1972, 1976, 1978), the Parent Counselors program in Alberta (Larson, Allison, & Johnston, 1978), the Parent Therapist program in Ontario (Levin, Rubenstein, & Streiner, 1976), and the Family Placement program in Kent, England (Hazel, 1981). These programs were forerunners of the 157 programs we have recently identified in Canada and the United States (Nutter, Hudson & Galaway, 1988) and which have also emerged in England and other parts of the world.

The papers in this volume identify important matters for consideration as we refine, develop, and expand this form of service. In this concluding chapter we consider five matters—variation among program approaches, social worker and foster parent roles, the role of birth parents, the relation of specialist foster care programming to permanency planning, and future directions for program development.

CONTRASTING MODELS

Agreement is emerging around some key features of specialized family care. Services are provided by families within their homes;

families are recruited and trained to provide the necessary care and
receive payment for services; social workers and other professional
staff provide supervision and consultation to the families who are
the primary service providers. There is agreement that families can
be recruited, trained, and supervised to provide care for very challenging children and youth who might otherwise be placed in institutional settings. Serving youth and children within the context of
families provides for flexibility in designing and carrying out individualized service plans. These papers suggest, however, that two
different approaches to specialized foster care may be emerging.

The papers by Pamela Meadowcroft and by Brad Bryant and his
colleagues refer to treatment within the foster home setting, while
Juanita Baker describes an educational program designed to train
foster parents to be "therapeutic change agents" with foster parents
taught to implement a child's written treatment plan designed by
outside professionals. The plan is to specify daily objectives for the
young person and a prescribed treatment routine followed within
the home. The service is referred to as treatment foster care with the
implication that treatment foster homes are a form of residential
treatment for one or two children. The picture is one of the institutional program having been implemented within the foster home.
Meadowcroft, for example, suggests that treatment foster care
should be thought of as the best of residential care.

A somewhat different approach is found in the papers by Hazel,
Smith, Peterson, Kelley and Carruth, Sisto and Maker, Kaplan and
Fein, and Hudson, Galaway, and Harmon. These authors tend to
emphasize concepts of normalization, youth participation in decision making, and viewing problems of youth from a perspective
which emphasizes young people interacting with their environments. This perspective comes out of an ecological framework with
a focus on developing a supportive environment and network of
social ties for the youth. Assisting youth with the work of dealing
responsibly with environments is the focus of concern; service
agreements address the reciprocal rights and responsibilities taken
on by young persons and significant persons with whom they interact. Foster parents are expected to serve as an advocate for youth,
help discover community resources, and assist young persons in
placement to become connected to their social environments.

These two approaches may indicate different historic roots for specialized foster family care. One may be from residential treatment centers or other residential mental health facilities that are shifting from institutional to family-based treatment services while at the same time maintaining much of the structure and self-containedness of the residential facility. An alternative root is out of traditional foster care. These may be two distinct approaches or a continuum of services. We may expect to find a wide range of ideas emerging regarding specialized foster care with program components mixed and matched as a considerable variety of service models respond to different populations and differing individuals.

FOSTER PARENT AND SOCIAL WORK ROLES

Mary McColgan notes ambivalence among social workers in traditional foster care programs about dealing with foster parents as colleagues or clients. This ambivalence is resolved in specialized foster family care programs. The authors agree that foster parents are professional colleagues of social workers, are the primary service providers, and function as full members of a service or treatment team. Emily Jean McFadden, for example, describes the need for a working alliance between foster parents and therapists in providing services to sexually abused children, while Susan Downs notes that the role of foster parents providing care for physically handicapped or developmentally disabled children must be reconceptualized to one of a professional service provider. In these chapters, McFadden and her colleagues define the mutually supportive roles of foster parents, social workers, and therapists working to prepare older foster children to emancipate from the foster home; Peter Smith points to the role of foster parents maintaining contacts with the birth parents. Baker and colleagues, as well as Meadowcroft, discuss the importance of training foster parents for their responsibility as service providers. Rosen, a foster parent, provides a description of how she carries out responsibilities of providing treatment foster care for autistic children.

This notion of foster parents as primary service providers and as equal members of a service team are illustrated further in the articles describing specialized foster care programs by Grace Sisto and Myra Maker, Michael Peterson, Christopher Kelley and James Carruth, Joe Hudson and colleagues, and Reuben Orenstein. The roles of social worker and foster parent have been realigned in specialized foster family care programs. Foster parents may take on duties often performed by social workers such as maintaining contact with birth parents and communication with schools and other community agencies on behalf of the child in placement. This presumes that foster parents will be fully informed about the young persons coming into their homes and will be consulted and involved in aftercare planning. The role of the social worker in specialized foster family care programs will shift away from direct service provision to team facilitation and supervision for foster parents.

ROLE OF THE BIRTH PARENTS

The role of birth parents in specialized foster family care scheme receives limited attention in these papers. Peter Forsythe calls for family-connectedness in all service planning. Ziona Kaplan and Edith Fein propose that foster parents serve as role models for birth parents to assist them in learning parenting skills, and Clarice Rosen, a foster parent, notes that foster parents must work closely with birth parents if consistency of response to autistic children is to be achieved. Brian Charbonneau and Ziona Kaplan describe the use of support and educational groups to engage and empower birth parents. Peter Smith makes the argument that involving birth parents with youth is essential to assist the young persons with identity formation and believes that birth parents should be involved in placement planning, including meeting foster families prior to placement. Nancy Hazel includes birth parents as co-equal partners in the service plan and thinks of foster parents as working partners with birth parents. The contracting process described by Joe Hudson, Burt Galaway, and Pat Harmon includes birth parents as participating members of the service team to develop and monitor service plans.

Specialized foster family care programs may need to give more attention to ways of empowering and involving birth parents in program activities. Should birth parents be routinely involved in pre-placement visits in the foster home? Should plans and procedures be put in place to provide for regular telephone and personal visits between birth parents and foster parents? Should birth parents, along with foster parents, be involved in key activities relating to the child in placement, such as attending school conferences, accompanying the child for medical visits, and celebrating important events in the life of the young person? Can birth parents join the foster parent-social worker team and be active participants in developing plans for and with their children? Conscious efforts and careful planning are necessary to avoid ignoring or leaving birth parents out of key decisions made about their children. In this way, specialized foster family care programs may carry out joint parenting in which two families, foster and birth, are involved jointly in the difficult task of rearing challenging children.

RELATION TO PERMANENCY PLANNING

The relationship of specialized foster family care to permanency planning has also received limited discussion among these papers. Peter Forsythe argues that family connectedness is important whether or not young people return to their birth parents. Peter Smith makes a similar argument based on the identity development needs of young persons. Kaplan and Fein as well as Charbonneau and Kaplan believe that specialized foster family care programs may assist young people to return to their birth parents as the permanent plan. Kelley and Carruth believe that many of the young people coming into treatment foster care programs will not be able to return home, and McFadden, Rice, Ryan, and Warren discuss the importance of preparing young people for emancipation from foster care.

Specialized foster family care is a resource for very difficult young people, often from very disorganized families who have not been responsive to intensive in-home services. This raises the very real possibility that specialized foster family care may become the permanent placement for some of these young people. Perhaps we need to expand our views about what is an appropriate permanency plan to include options beyond adoption or return home. Many of these youth may require the stability and highly skilled services of specialized foster homes to mature into adulthood. This does not, of course, deny the young person opportunities to be involved with birth parents and will involve a joint-parenting arrangement in which the young person is assured stable placement in a specialized foster family home while regularly interacting with birth parents who participate in key care decisions. Such a plan provides a stable living arrangement and opportunities to maintain and strengthen links with the birth family.

Another aspect of permanency planning is the matter of continuing contact between foster parents, the youth, and birth parents when the youth has returned home. The foster parents will have played an important role in the life of the young person and perhaps with the birth parents and will have established close bonds of mutual respect and affection. We must question, therefore, the rationale for sharply limiting or curtailing contacts between foster parents and the youth when the youth has returned home. Should not continuing contact and communication be encouraged and made formal with specific plans developed to facilitate communication? The papers by Hazel and McFadden and colleagues note that emancipated foster children need continuing support from their foster parents, just like most young people who have left home. Might this not also hold true for young people who have returned to live with birth parents? If the birth parents have been appropriately involved in planning during the placement and the concept of joint parenting was operationalized, would they not also enjoy and benefit from the continued support of contacts with the foster parents?

FUTURE DIRECTIONS

The papers in this volume provide illustrations of the use of specialized family care with diverse and challenging children and youth. McFadden discusses use of specialized foster family care with sexually abused children and Downs with mentally retarded and physically handicapped. Rosen provides a case illustration of treatment foster care for autistic children, Sisto and Maker illustrate the use of specialized foster family care for teenage mothers and their babies, and Kelley and Carruth with delinquent youth. Smith and Hazel's work describes a program for both delinquent and disturbed adolescents; papers by Meadowcroft, Peterson, Orenstein, and Hudson, Galaway, and Harmon all describe specialized foster family programs for a variety of disturbed children and youth. Specialized foster family care programs are likely to continue to develop for several reasons—lower cost than residential treatment, broadened acceptance of the principle of least restrictive alternative, recognition that family-centered care will more successfully prepare persons for adulthood and citizenship than institutional care, flexibility to develop individual plans to meet specific needs of children and youth, and avoiding the damaging effects of intrusiveness and regimentation of institutional settings.

We expect the number of specialized foster family care programs to increase rapidly. Along with the growth in number we expect several different treatment or service models to emerge and become more distinct. The papers in this volume illustrate programs developed by public agencies (McColgan; Bryant, Simmens, & McKee; Smith; Orenstein), nonprofit social agencies (Kaplan & Fein; Sisto & Maker; Peterson; Kelley & Carruth), and for-profit social agencies (Hudson, Galaway, & Harmon). Program development will continue in all three sectors with the private sector continuing to lead the way. The ability of private agencies to concentrate on a single programming thrust along with the already well-established private delivery of specialized foster family care suggests more active program development by private businesses, nonprofit and for profit, than by government. Government will continue to be the major purchaser of the service.

Specialized foster family care services will also be extended to additional populations, especially adults. The article by Leigh Jones illustrates the use of family placement as an alternative to institutional placement for aged persons. Family care may well provide a resource for other older people, including developmentally disabled, mentally ill, and offenders. Specialized foster family homes may be used, for example, for adult female offenders and their children and for adult offenders on work release as an alternative to jails.

Specialized foster family care may become a cottage industry in which couples pursue a career and make a living providing family-centered care within their own homes. In time we expect to see the end of the term foster parent as support coalesces around one of the other terms beginning to emerge such as foster carer, foster care provider, community care provider, or something similar. Whatever title emerges, the central concept of providing family-centered care rather than institutional care will continue to develop and to expand. We recognize, in the words of Nancy Hazel, that "no person is unsuitable for family placement, although it may not be possible to provide the family environment which would be suitable for particular people." The future will provide an increasing number of these family environments.

References

Allegheny County Children and Youth Services (1987). *Draft plan update and budget estimate for 1988 and 1989 for children and youth and child protective services*. Pittsburgh, PA: Allegheny County Children and Youth Services.

Amara, R. (1979). An overview on the social responsibility of business. In A. Starchild (Ed.), *Business in 1990* (pp. 52-65). Seattle: University Press of the Pacific.

Anderson, J., & Simonitch, B. (1981). Reactive depression in youths experiencing emancipation. *Child Welfare*, *60*(6), 383-390.

Appathurai, C., Lowery, G., & Sullivan, T. (1986). Achieving the vision of deinstitutionalization: A role for foster care? *Child and Adolescent Social Work*, *3*.

Arcari, M., & Betman, B. (1986). The deaf child in foster care. *Children Today*, *15*(4), 17-21.

Armstrong, K. A. (1981). A treatment and education program for parents and children who are at risk of abuse and neglect. *Child Abuse and Neglect*, *5*(2), 167-175.

Baldwin, W., & Cain, V. (1980, January/February). The children of teenage parents. *Family Planning Perspectives*, *12*(1), 34-44.

Barnado's (n.d.). *Proposed extension of professional foster home scheme*. Unpublished paper on Barnado's Professional Foster Care Project.

Barnado's Professional Foster Care Project (1985). Unpublished paper.

Barnett, B. (1985, October 4-5). Foster kids speak up: Help us. *The Children's Chronicle*. St. Louis, MO.

Barth, R. (1986). Emancipation services for adolescents in foster care. *Social Work*, *31*(3), 165-171.

Beck, A. T. (1976). *Cognitive theory and the emotional disorders*. New York: International University Press.

Becker, W. C. (1971). *Parents are teachers*. Champaign, IL: Research Press.

Behan, B. (1958). *Borstal boy*. London: Huchinson.

Bennis, W. G., Benne, K. D., Chin, R., & Corey, K. E. (1976). *The planning of change* [3rd ed.]. New York: Holt, Rinehart and Winston.

Birrel, D., & Murie, A. (1981). *Policy and government in Northern Ireland*. London: Gill and Macmillan.

Blom-Cooper, L. (1985). *A child in trust: The report of the panel of inquiry into the circumstances surrounding the death of Jasmine Beckford*. Brent: London Borough Council and Brent Health Authority.

Bolton, R. (1979). *People skills, how to assert yourself, listen to others, and resolve conflicts*. Englewood Cliffs, NJ: Prentice-Hall, Inc.

Boyd, L. H., & Remy, L. L. (1979). Foster parents who stay licensed and the role of training. *Journal of Social Service Research, 2*(4), 478-490.

Brandt, R., & Tisza, V. (1979). The sexually misused child. *American Journal of Orthopsychiatry, 49*(1), 80-90.

Braukmann, C. J., Fixsen, D. L., Kirigin, K. A., Phillips, E. A., Phillips, E. L., & Wolf, M. M. (1975). Achievement place: The training and certification of teaching parents. In W. S. Wood (Ed.), *Issues in evaluating behavior modification*. Champaign, IL: Research Press.

Bruggen, P., & Pitt-Aiken, T. (1975). Authority as a key factor in adolescent disturbance. *British Journal of Medical Psychology, 48*, Part 2, 153-159.

Bryant, B. (1983). *Integrative management in new breed organization*. Staunton, VA: People Places, Inc.

Bryant, B. (1981). Special foster care: A history and rationale. *Journal of Clinical Child Psychology, 10*(1), 8-20.

Bryant, B. (1980). *Special foster care: A history and rationale*. Staunton, VA: People Places, Inc.

Bryant, B. (1984). *Special foster care: Evaluation of an alternative to institutions for disturbed children*. Unpublished master's thesis, University of Virginia, Charlottesville.

Burge, D., Fabry, B., Conoway, R., & James, J. (1987). Meeting

the challenge: Treating diverse and difficult problems in therapeutic foster families. In P. Meadowcroft & C. Almeida
(Chairs), *Foster parents as treatment agents*. Symposium presented at the American Psychological Association Convention,
New York City, NY.

Campbell, C., & Downs, S. W. (1987). The impact of economic
incentives in fostering. *Social Service Review*, *61*(4), 599-609.

Carros, T., & Kriksten, D. (in press). A public child welfare
agency view of special foster care and foster family-based treatment. In R. P. Hawkins & J. Brieling (Eds.), *Treatment parenting: Issues in development, evaluation, and dissemination*.
Washington, DC: Child Welfare League of America.

Cautley, P. W. (1980). *New foster parents: The first experience*.
New York: Human Sciences Press.

Central Personal Social Services Advisory Committee (1980). *Report of the sub-committee on foster care in Northern Ireland*.
Belfast: Department of Health and Social Services.

Charpie, R. (1979). Intermediate institutions. In A. Starchild (Ed.),
Business in 1990 (pp. 132-145). Seattle: University Press of the
Pacific.

Chiaro, J., Marden, G., Haase, L., & Guedes, B. (1982, September). *Mismatching of the foster parents and the sexually abused
pre-school child*. Paper presented at the 4th International Conference on Child Abuse and Neglect, Paris, France.

Children and Young Persons Review Group (1977). *Legislation
and services for children and young persons in N. Ireland*. Belfast: HMSO.

Chilman, C. (Ed.) (1980). Adolescent pregnancy and childbearing.
Washington, DC: US Government Printing Office.

Clark, L. (1985). *SOS! Help for parents*. Bowling Green, KY: Parents Press.

Colon, F. (1973). In search of one's past: An identity trip. *Family
Process*, *12*(4), 429-438.

Comfort, R. (1985). Sex, strangers and safety. *Child Welfare*,
64(5), 541-546.

Cousins, J. (1983). *The need for independent living in the foster
care system*. Paper presented at Regional Youth conference, La-
kewood, OH.

Coyne, A. (1986). Recruiting foster and adoptive families: A marketing strategy. *Children Today*, *15*(5), 30-33.

Craigavon, the Decision Partnership (1978). *Report of the Royal Commission of the National Health Service on the management of financial resources in the National Health Service with particular reference to Northern Ireland.*

Cunningham, M. (1982). *Helping the sexually abused child.* Marin County, CA: Marin County Department of Health and Human Services.

Damon, L., Todd, J., & McFarlane, K. (1987). Treatment issues with sexually abused young children. *Child Welfare*, *66*(2), 123-137.

Dawson, R. (1985). *T.R.U.S.T. II: Fostering sexually abused children.* Oxford: Ontario Ministry of Community and Social Services.

Davis, A. B., Foster, P. H., & Whitworth, F. M. (1984). Medical foster family care: A cost effective solution to a community problem. *Child Welfare*, *63*(4), 341-351.

Deal, T. E., & Kennedy, A. A. (1982). *Corporate cultures: The rites and rituals of corporate life.* Reading, MA: Addison-Wesley.

DeJong, G. (1975). Setting foster care rates: 1. Basic considerations. *Public Welfare*, *33*(4), 37-41.

Department of Health and Social Security (1987). *The law on child care and family services.* London: HMSO.

DeWeaver, L. (1983). Deinstitutionalization of the developmentally disabled. *Social Work*, *28*(6), 435-439.

Dickens, C. (1838). *Oliver Twist or the parish boy's progress* (Quoted from 1986 London, Penguin reprint, p. 56). London: R. Bentley.

Dixon, J., & Jenkin, J. O. (1981). Incestuous child abuse: A review of treatment strategies. *Clinical Psychology Review*, *1*(2), 211-222.

Downs, S. W. (1989). Foster parents of teenagers: Special parents, special needs. In A. Maluccio, R. Krieger, & B. Pine (Eds.), *Preparing for life after foster care: The central role of foster parents.* Washington: Child Welfare League of America.

Eddy, W. B. (1982). Organization development and change. In F.

S. Lane (Ed.), *Current issues in public administration* (pp. 265-280). New York: St. Martin's Press.

Ellis, A. (1962). *Reason and emotion in psychotherapy*. New York: Lyle Stuart.

Erikson, E. H. (1959). *Identity and the life cycle*. New York: International Universities Press.

Erikson, E. H. (1968). *Identity, youth and crisis*. New York: Norton.

Euster, S., Ward, V., Varner, J., & Euster, G. (1984). Life skills group for adolescent foster children. *Child Welfare*, *63*(1), 27-36.

Evason, E. (1976). *Social need and social provision in North Ireland*. Coleraine: New University of Ulster.

Fabry, B., Meadowcroft, P., Frost, S., Hawkins, R. P., & Conoway, R. (1987). Low cost, high validity, multi-use data: Practical program evaluation in a family-based treatment program. Paper presented at the Association of Behavior Analysis Convention, Nashville, TN.

Fabry, B., & James, M. J. (1985). Aggressive youths. Workshop presentation at the West Virginia Therapeutic Foster Care Conference, Charleston, WV.

Fanshel, D., & Shinn, E. B. (1978). *Children in foster care: A longitudinal investigation*. New York: Columbia University Press.

Festinger, T. (1983). *No one ever asked us: A postscript to foster care*. New York: Columbia University Press.

Fisher, M., Marsh, P., & Phillips, D. with E. E. Sainsbury. (1986). *In and out of care: The experiences of children, parents, and social workers*. London: Batsford.

Fleischman, M. J., Horne, A. M., & Arthur, J. L. (1983). *Troubled families treatment program*. Champaign, IL: Research Press Co.

Foster, P. H., & Whitmore, J. M. (1986). Medical foster care: An alternative to long-term hospitalization. *Children Today*, *15*(4), 12-16.

Furrh, P. (1983). Emancipation: The supervised apartment living approach. *Child Welfare*, *62*(1), 54-61.

Galaway, B. (1978). PATH: An agency operated by foster parents. *Child Welfare, 57*(10), 667-674.

Galaway, B. (1976). Contracting: A means of clarifying roles in foster family services. *Children Today, 5*(4), 20-23.

Galaway, B. (1972). Clarifying the role of foster parents. *Children Today, 1*(4), 32-33.

Galbraith, J. K. (1967). *The new industrial state.* Boston: Houghton-Mifflin.

Geiser, R. (1973). *The illusion of caring: Children in foster care.* Boston: Brown Press.

Gideon, S. (1986). The Parent Therapist Program. Workshop presentation at CASSP/NIMH Conference, Boulder, CO.

Gil, E., & Bogart, K. (1982). Foster children speak out. *Children Today, 11*(1), 7-9.

Golembiewski, R. T., & Eddy, W. B. (1978). *Organization development in public administration.* New York: Marcel Dekker.

Gordon, T. (1970). *P.E.T. parent effectiveness training.* New York: Peter H. Wyden, Inc.

Goss, D. (1986). *Treatment foster families: A study of family adaptability through crises events.* Unpublished senior thesis, Chatham College, Pittsburgh, PA.

Goss, G. (1987). Personal communication to Pam Meadowcroft.

Grealish, E. M., Hunt, J., Lynch, P. J., & James, M. J. (1987). Professional parent recruitment: Effective methods for family-based treatment programs. Paper presented at the Southeast Psychology Association Convention, Atlanta, GA.

Griffin, W. (1985). *Independent living strategies.* Chapel Hill, NC: National Child Welfare Leadership Center.

Gruber, A. (1978). *Children in foster care, destitute, neglected, betrayed.* New York: Human Sciences Press.

Haley, J. (1980). *Leaving home.* New York: McGraw-Hill.

Harbinson, J. (1983). *Children of the troubles.* Belfast: Stranmillis College.

Hardin, M., & Tazzara, P. (1983). *Foster parents rights to share in decision-making for the foster child.* Washington, DC: American Bar Association.

Hawkins, R. P., & Luster, W. C. (1982). Foster family-based treatment: A minimally restrictive alternative with special promise.

Paper presented at the American Psychological Association Convention, Washington, DC.

Hawkins, R. P., & Meadowcroft, P. (1984). *Practical program evaluation in a foster family-based treatment program for disturbing and disturbed youngsters*. Pittsburgh, PA: Pressley Ridge Schools.

Hawkins, R. P., Meadowcroft, P., Trout, B. A., & Luster, W. C. (1985). Foster family-based treatment. *Journal of Clinical Child Psychology, 14*(3), 220-228.

Hazel, N. (1981). *A bridge to independence*. Oxford: Blackwell.

Herron, S., & Caul, B. (1980). *A service for people: Origins and development of the personal social services of Northern Ireland*. Belfast: Ulster Polytechnic.

Hoghughi, M. (1985). *Towards a disciple of fostering*. London: National Foster Care Association.

Horesji, C. (1979). *Foster family care*. Springfield, IL: Charles C. Thomas.

Horejsi, R. (1979). Developmental disabilities: Opportunities for social workers. *Social Work, 24*(1), 40-45.

House of Commons. *Second report from the social services committee, session 1983-84, children in care*. [para. 171]. London: HMSO.

Jones, E. F., Forrest, J. D., Goldman, N., Henshaw, S. K., Lincoln, R., Rosoff, J. I., Westoff, C. F., & Wulf, D. (1985). Teenage pregnancy in developed countries: Determinants and policy implications. *Family Planning Perspectives, 17*(2), 53-63.

Jones, M. A., & Moses, B. (1984). *West Virginia's former foster children: Their experiences in care and their lives as young adults*. New York: Child Welfare League of America.

Jordan, M. (1986, July 20). Foster parent scarcity causing crisis in care. *Washington Post*, F1 & F8.

Justice, B., & Justice, R. (1979). *The broken taboo: Sex in the family*. New York: Human Sciences.

Kanfer, F. H. (1975). Self-management methods. In F. H. Kanfer and A. P. Goldstein (Eds.), *Helping people change*. New York: Pergamon Press.

Kelly, B. (1979). Social work in Northern Ireland. *Social Work Today*, *10*(27), pp. 16-22.

Kent Family Placement Service. (1985) *Ten years on—a pioneer teenage fostering scheme, 1975 to 1985*. Maidstone: Kent County Council.

Kerr, M. E. (1981). Family systems, theory and therapy. In A. Gurman & D. Knisken (Eds.), *Handbook of family therapy*. New York: Brunnau/Mazel, Inc.

Kirgan, D. (1983). Meeting children's needs through placement. *Child Welfare*, *63*(2), 157-166.

Kirigin, K. A., Braukmann, C. J., Atwater, J. D., & Wolf, M. M. (1982). An evaluation of teaching family group homes for juvenile offenders. *Journal of Applied Behavior Analysis*, *15*(1), 1-16.

Kriegish, L., Richardson, M., Lichtenfels, W., Lilley, J., Fabry, B., & Hawkins, R. P. (1986). *The Pressley Ridge Schools followup project: PRYDE report*. Pittsburgh, PA; Pressley Ridge Schools.

Laird, J. (1978). Ecologically oriented child welfare practice: Issues of family identity and continuity. In C. Germain (Ed.), *Social work practice: People and environments* (pp. 178-209). New York: Columbia University Press.

Larson, G., Allison, J., & Johnston, E. (1978). Alberta parent counselors: A community treatment program for disturbed youths. *Child Welfare*, *57*(1), 47-52.

Levin, S., Rubenstein, J., & Streiner, D. (1976). The parent therapist program: An innovative approach to treating emotionally disturbed children. *Hospital and Community Psychiatry*, *27*(6), 407-410.

Littner, N. (1956). *Some traumatic effects of separation and placement*. New York: Child Welfare League of America.

Littner, N. (1960). The child's need to repeat his past: Some implications for placement. *Social Services Review*, *34*(2), 128-148.

Maluccio, A. N. (1985). *Improving the ability of foster parents to help near emancipated youth: Innovative curriculum materials, training tools and training methods*. West Hartford: University of Connecticut School of Social Work.

Maluccio, A. N., & Fein, E. (1985). Growing up in foster care.

Children and Youth Services Review, 7, 123-134. Pergamon Press.

Maluccio, A. N., & Fein, E. (1983). Permanency planning: A redefinition. *Child Welfare*, 62(3), 195-201.

Maluccio, A. N., Fein, E., Hamilton, V. J., Klier, J., & Ward, D. (1980). Beyond permanency planning. *Child Welfare*, 59(9), 515-530.

Maluccio, A. N., Fein, E., & Olmstead, K. A. (1986). *Permanency planning for children*. New York: Tavistock Publications.

Marron, S. et al. (1982). *Open door: An introduction to foster care in the Republic of Ireland*. Dublin: Irish Foster Care Association.

Maslow, A. H. (1954). *Motivation and personality*. New York: Harper.

McFadden, E. J. (1986). *Fostering the child who has been sexually abused*. Ypsilanti: Eastern Michigan University.

McFadden, E. J. (1985). Practice in foster care. In J. Laird & A. Hartman (Eds.), *Handbook of child welfare*. New York: Free Press.

McFadden, E. J. (1984a). *Emotional development*. Ypsilanti: Eastern Michigan University.

McFadden, E. J. (1984b). *Preventing abuse in foster care*. Ypsilanti: Eastern Michigan University.

McFadden, E. J., & Ryan, P. (1986, August). *Characteristics of the vulnerable child*. Paper presented at Sixth International Conference on Child Abuse and Neglect, Sydney, Australia.

McFadden, E. J., & Stovall, B. (1984). Child sexual abuse in family foster care. *Preventing abuse in foster care*. Ypsilanti: Eastern Michigan University.

Meadowcroft, P., & Grealish, E. M. (1985). Training and supporting treatment parents. In B. A. Trout & P. Meadowcroft (Eds.), *Troubled youths in treatment homes*. Pittsburgh, PA: Pressley Ridge Schools.

Meadowcroft, P. (1987, August). *Troubled youths in treatment homes*. Keynote address, First North American Treatment Foster Care Conference, Minneapolis, MN.

Meichenbaum, D. (1977). *Cognitive-behavior modification: An integrative approach*. New York: Plenum Press.

Miller, F. (1982). *Protection of children in foster family care*. New York: Vera Institute of Justice.

Miller, K., Fein, E., Howe, G., Gaudio, C., & Bishop, G. (1984). Time-limited goal-focused parent aide services. *Social Casework, 65*(8), 472-477.

Millham, S., Bullock, R., Hosie, K., & Haak, M. (1986). *Lost in care: The problems of maintaining links between children in care and their families*. Aldershot, England: Gower.

Mitchell, A. K. (1985). *Children in the middle: Living through divorce*. London: Tavistock.

Mrazek, P. B., & Kempe, C. H. (1981). *Sexually abused children and their families*. New York: Pergamon.

Nasjleti, M. (1980). Suffering in silence: The male incest victim. *Child Welfare, 59*(5), 269-275.

National Commission for Children in Need of Parents (1979). *Who knows, who cares? Forgotten children in foster care*. New York: Institute of Public Affairs.

Nigro, F. A., & Nigro, L. G. (1977). *Modern public administration* [4th ed.]. New York: Harper & Row.

Nova University (1978). *Pre-service foster parent training: A manual for trainers*. Fort Lauderdale, FL: Foster Parent Project, Nova University.

Nutter, R., Hudson, J., & Galaway, B. (1988). Specialist fostering: Results of a North American survey. Paper presented at the Second North American Treatment Foster Care Conference, Calgary, Alberta, August 3-5, 1988.

O'Dell, S. (1974). Training parents in behavior modification: A review. *Psychological Bulletin, 81*(7), 418.

Palazolli, M., Boscolo, L., Cecahin, G. F., & Prata, G. (1977). Family rituals: A powerful tool in family therapy. *Family Process, 16*, 445-453.

Pardeck, J. T. (1982). *The forgotten child: A study of the stability and continuity of foster care*. Washington, DC: University Press of America.

Parker, R. A. (1966). *Decision in child care*. London: Allen and Unwin.

Phillips, E. L., Phillips, E. A., Fixsen, D. L., & Wolf, M. M.

(1974). *The teaching family handbook*. Lawrence: University of Kansas Printing Service.

Piaget, J. Piaget's theory. In P. H. Mussen (Ed.), *Carmichael's Manual of Child Psychology* [3rd ed.] (pp. 703-732). New York: Wiley.

Pierce, J. (1987). *Summary report on the meeting of Pennsylvania therapeutic foster care programs*. Pennsylvania Council on Children Services, Harrisburg, PA.

Polsky, H. W. (1962). *Cottage Six*. New York: John Wiley.

Powell, F. (1980). The effect of the Northern Ireland civil conflict on child welfare. *International Social Work, 23*(2), 25-32.

Reasoner, R. W. (1982). *Building self-esteem: Administrator's guide*. Palo Alto, CA: Consulting Psychologists Press.

Reid, W. F., & Epstein, L. (1972). *Task-centered casework*. New York: Columbia University Press.

Reid, W. F. (1978). *The task-centered system*. New York: Columbia University Press.

Reitz, A. (1987). *Program report to the Pressley Ridge Schools Board of Trustees*. Pittsburgh, PA.

Rest, E., & Watson, K. (1984). Growing up in foster care. *Child Welfare, 63*(4), 291-304.

Rice, D., & Semmelroth, S. (1968). Foster care for emotionally disturbed children. *American Journal of Orthopsychiatry*, (April) 539-542.

Rowe, J. (1980). Fostering in the 1970's and beyond. In J. Triseliotis (Ed.), *New development in foster care and adoption*. London: Routledge Kegan Paul.

Rowe, J., Cain, H., Hundleby, M., & Keane, A. (1984). *Long term foster care*. London: Batsford.

Rowe, P. (1983). Bridging the gap from foster care to independent living. *Children Today, 12*(5), 28-29.

Ryan, P. (1983). Survey of abuse and neglect in foster care. *Impact*. Ypsilanti: Eastern Michigan University.

Ryan, P. (1978). *Issues in fostering*. Ypsilanti: Eastern Michigan University.

Sayles, L. R. (1979). *Leadership: What effective managers really do and how they do it*. New York: McGraw-Hill.

Selby, R. S. (1985). *Delinquency treatment: An evaluation of the*

Youth Advocate Program. Bowling Green State University, PhD dissertation. Ann Arbor, MI: University Microfilms.

Settles, B. H., Van Name, J. B., & Culley, J. D. (1976). Estimating costs in foster family care. *Children Today*, 5(6), 19ff.

Shapiro, D. (1970). *Agencies and foster children*. New York: Columbia University Press.

Shaw, M., & Hipgrave, T. (1983). *Specialist Fostering*. London: Batsford Academic and Educational Ltd.

Simon, J. L. (1975). The effect of foster care payment levels on the number of foster children given homes. *Social Service Review*, 49, 405-411.

Simonitch, B., & Anderson, J. L. (1979). On their own: An Oregon Experiment. *Children Today*, 8(5).

Smith, R. (1984). *Adoption and fostering*. London: Macmillan.

Snodgrass, R. D., & Bryant, B. (1984). *Special foster care: Past and present*. Staunton, VA: People Places, Inc.

Southern Health and Social Services Board. (1987). Fee-paid placement scheme. Unpublished paper.

Specht, C. (1975). Setting foster care rates: 2. Special cases. *Public Welfare*, 33(4), 42-46.

Stein, T. J., Gambrill, E. D., & Wiltse, K. T. (1978). *Children in foster homes: Achieving continuity of care*. New York: Praeger Publishers.

Stepleton, S. (1987). Specialized foster care: Families as treatment resources. *Children Today*, 16(2), 27-31.

Stroul, B. A., & Friedman, R. M. (1986). *A system of care for seriously emotionally disturbed children and youth*. Washington, DC: CASSP Technical Assistance Center at Georgetown University.

Stroul, B. A., & Goldman, S. (in preparation). A national study of in home services, therapeutic foster care, and crisis intervention for seriously emotionally disturbed children. CASSP Technical Assistance Center, Georgetown University.

Tatara, T., & Pettiford, E. K. (1986). *Characteristics of children in substitute and adoptive care: A statistical summary of the VCIS National Child Welfare Data Base*. Washington, DC: American Public Welfare Association.

Therapeutic foster care. (1986). *Update*, 2(1), 8-10.

Tinney, M. A. (1985). Role perceptions in foster parent associations in British Columbia. *Child Welfare*, *64*(1), 73-79.

Toffler, A. (1980). *The third wave*. New York: William Morrow.

Tooley, K. (1978). The remembrance of things past: On the collection and recollection of ingredients useful in the treatment of disorder resulting from unhappiness, rootlessness, and the fear of things to come. *American Journal of Orthopsychiatry*, *48*(1), 174-182.

Tremitiere, B. T. (1979). Adoption of children with special needs: The client centered approach. *Child Welfare*, *58*(10), 681-685.

Trout, B. A. (1985). *PRYDE discharge data*. Pittsburgh, PA: Pressley Ridge Schools.

Trout, B. A., & Meadowcroft, P. (1985). *Troubled youths in treatment homes*. Pittsburgh, PA: Pressley Ridge Schools.

U.S. Congress, Office of Technology Assessment. (1986). *Children's mental health problems and services*. Washington, DC: Government Printing Office.

Vera Institute of Justice (1981). *Foster home child protection*. New York: Human Resources Administration.

Vernon, J., & Fruin, D. (1985). *In care: A study of social work decision making*. London: National Children's Bureau.

Vincent, C. (1961). *Unmarried mothers*. New York: Free Press.

Virginia Department of Social Services (1986). *Report of task force on the status of older children in foster care*. Richmond: Commonwealth of Virginia.

Wallerstein, J. S., & Kelly, J. B. (1980). *Surviving the break-up: How children and parents cope with divorce*. London: Grant McIntyre.

Wilkes, D. (1974). The impact of fostering on the foster family. *Child Welfare*, *53*(6), 373-379.

Working Party on Fostering Practice (1976). *A guide to fostering practice*. London: HMSO.

Young, L. (154). *Out of wedlock*. New York: McGraw-Hill.